Interpreting
CT Head Scans

Dedicated to
The Radiology staff at The Queen Elizabeth Hospital;
to Ros, Michael and David
and
Stan

Interpreting CT Head Scans

A basic guide to image analysis

Lynda E. Albertyn
FRACR
Senior Visiting Specialist

Randell V. Brown
FRACR
Senior Visiting Specialist

Department of Radiology
The Queen Elizabeth Hospital
Woodville
South Australia

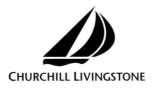

CHURCHILL LIVINGSTONE

NEW YORK, EDINBURGH, LONDON, MADRID, MELBOURNE, SAN FRANCISCO AND TOKYO 1996

CHURCHILL LIVINGSTONE
Medical Division of Pearson Professional Limited

Distributed in the United States of America by Churchill
Livingstone Inc., 650 Avenue of the Americas, New York,
N.Y. 10011, and by associated companies, branches and
representatives throughout the world.

© Pearson Professional Limited 1996

First published 1996

ISBN 0 443 05029 5

British Library Cataloguing in Publication Data
A catalogue record for this book is available from the British
Library.

Library of Congress Cataloging in Publication Data
A catalog record for this book is available from the Library of
Congress.

For Churchill Livingstone:

Publisher: Geoff Nuttall
Editor: Gavin Smith
Design: Sarah Cape
Production: Anita Sekhri

Produced by Longman Singapore Publishers (Pte) Ltd
Printed in Singapore

The
publisher's
policy is to use
**paper manufactured
from sustainable forests**

ACKNOWLEDGEMENTS

We wish to thank our friends and colleagues at our hospital and in our local professional community, including the neurologists and neurosurgeons who willingly allowed us to assemble the teaching material for the library from which this book is drawn.

We thank Manohar Hullan for his illustrations; Jim Antoniou for his computer assistance; Alex Hetman and Paula Gallasch for their exquisite photography; Geoff West our senior CT radiographer for his intelligent professionalism; Ruben Sebben for his radiologic excellence and his maverick humour; Heather Webber for being a good friend and colleague; Bill Tucker for his forthright mentorship; and Doreen Marks who smiled as she typed.

We acknowledge a long line of CT fellows from all over Australasia who, by repeatedly asking similar questions, showed us what radiologists needed to learn in order to gain initial confidence in CT interpretation. Our registrars in training, and many in neurology, neurosurgery, psychiatry, and internal medicine reinforced this thinking, and we thank them too.

PREFACE

This book was conceived as a simple practical introduction to cranial CT, which we believe is now firmly in the domain of the general radiologist, and no longer the preserve of the dedicated neuroradiologist. Work pattern analysis in any large hospital or practice will show what a major contribution cranial CT makes to everyday work, and what a high percentage of after-hours emergencies require CT, often with relatively junior medical staff in the first line of call. CT has revolutionized the entire modern approach to trauma and all other acute neurologic presentations. In smaller centres CT is used as a cost-effective critical triaging step in deciding where patients should be managed. Psychiatrists can now exclude with more confidence the possibility of treatable organic disease in their patients and hope for an improved understanding of disease in others, and for neurosurgeons the visual correlation with the macropathology they will encounter is revolutionary.

For all of us there have been perceptual, geometric and analytic challenges in coming to grips with 'slice' imaging. Image quality is now so good that much of the uncertainty associated with the original rather crude pictures has been eliminated.

We have deliberately chosen an approach which is independent of the level of sophistication of the CT scanner used, and have therefore not discussed spiral, dynamic or any of the other scanning refinements now available. In clinical practice, the emphasis still remains on reading the final image and, provided it is good, it doesn't matter how it has been generated. The section on physics and techniques has been kept as simple as possible, with the emphasis on aspects like slice thickness, windowing, Hounsfield values and the role of intravenous contrast. The anatomy section likewise has been designed to help readers know what structures they might reasonably hope to identify, and practical clinical points and correlations run through the text.

In the section on the interpretation of the abnormal scan, which forms the bulk of the book, the emphasis is on dissection of the image along the lines of a few useful principles which will be informative about the nature and urgency of the pathophysiology involved. If the image can be broken down this way we believe broad diagnostic categories can be reached and sensible management decisions made.

No attempt has been made to include detailed or uncommon neuropathology. There are many excellent comprehensive texts which already do this. Where lists of possible diagnoses are included they have been designed to emphasize common and important conditions and to put these in clinical perspective.

Other than the anatomical drawings, the illustrations have been confined to CT, even when it was tempting to include other imaging, especially magnetic resonance. For many diagnosticians and clinicians around the world, CT will still be the first line of investigation, and we believe that the three-dimensional integration approach, the search patterns and the recognition of pathophysiological mechanisms which one can learn from CT are readily translatable to magnetic resonance. The picture may change, but the pathology remains the same.

CONTENTS

Contents

CHAPTER 1

Introduction

This book is not meant to be a comprehensive guide to pathology or an atlas from which one can make visual matches. Instead, it is designed to emphasize the principles involved in image analysis in CT, based on the old Chinese proverb that if you give a man a fish, he eats for the day, but if you teach him how to fish, he eats for the rest of his life.

The prime requirement is obviously the generation of a good image. The first section on Physics deals with this. Once a good image has been generated it must be displayed and photographed appropriately.

Armed with some basic anatomic knowledge, the next step is to assess the physical basis of any lesion which disturbs the normal symmetry of the intracranial contents. This will involve observations such as whether the lesion is single or multiple, focal or diffuse, space occupying or space creating and so forth.

Every additional objective observation strengthens the macropathological description and narrows the field of possible diagnoses still further.

Pattern recognition is the origin of the term 'Aunt Minnie'. One may recognize Aunt Minnie immediately if she is the only person one knows. This is beginner's luck. Generally speaking, however, one's recognition of Aunt Minnie is enhanced by the ability to recognize multiple physical characteristics of Aunt Minnie which, in combination, virtually exclude the possibility that she could be anyone else. With experience, this recognition becomes very rapid. This can be an impressive performance but one which is difficult to communicate to an apprentice.

It is therefore more useful to teach systematic image analysis by emphasizing the following key questions.

Key questions in approaching cranial CT

1. Where is the lesion?
2. What is its shape?
3. What is its physical composition?
4. How does it behave with intravenous contrast?
5. How does it behave with gravity?
6. How does it behave with time?

In combination, the answer to these questions will frequently bring one close to a specific diagnosis.

The book is an application of these principles, based on many enjoyable and entertaining years' experience in introducing people to the elegant potential of CT.

Bibliography

Andreasen N C 1992 Neuroradiology and neuro-psychiatry: a new alliance. American Journal of Roentgenology 13: 841–843

CHAPTER 2

Physics and scanning principles

i. Historical perspective

In the 1970s Computerized Tomography revolutionized imaging of the human body. From its inception CT's ability to provide direct information about the existence and nature of intracranial pathology was quickly appreciated and made the indirect imaging techniques such as ventriculography obsolete.

Godfrey Hounsfield, an English scientist working in the research department of EMI, is commonly regarded as the father of CT. Workers in Russia, Japan and other countries had been working for decades on the concept of cross-sectional body imaging, but it was the research and development undertaken by Hounsfield and his team between 1967 and 1970 which resulted in the first clinically useful scanner being installed at the Atkinson–Morley Hospital, Wimbledon in London in 1971. Hounsfield and Ambrose presented the first paper on CT to the British Institute of Radiography in 1972, and the importance of their work was immediately recognized.

The original EMI scanner took 6 minutes to perform one slice and 20 minutes to reconstruct the image. New generations of scanners using advanced computer technology, fan X-ray beams and multiple detectors have enabled single slices to be performed in as little as two seconds with virtually immediate image reconstruction. The technology is available to perform scans in milliseconds but these scanners are not yet commonly used in clinical practice.

CT is now regarded by many as the linchpin of modern diagnostic imaging. Its constant value in many clinical situations, as well as its relative simplicity in operation and interpretation, has demystified it and made it indispensable to most modern diagnostic units.

ii. Basic physical principles

The internal structure of an object can be reconstructed from multiple projections of the object. For example, a simple mathematical puzzle uses this principle to solve for a, b, c and d.

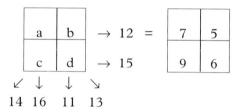

With CT, an image of a body slice is obtained by taking a very large number of narrow X-ray beam projections at multiple angles through that slice. Assuming the intensity of the X-ray beam as it enters the body is constant, then measurement of the intensity of the emerging beam will reflect the magnitude of the absorption of X-rays by the body. This varies depending primarily on tissue density, and is readily analogous to the differential absorption used in conventional radiology. This is easily appreciated by anybody who has pondered a chest X-ray. If sufficient pencil beam X-ray projections of a single slice are taken, mathematical analysis will yield an image of that slice (Fig. 2.1).

Hardware

A CT scanner consists of an X-ray tube and detector array mounted on opposite sides of the patient on a rigid gantry and contained within a doughnut-shaped jacket. Original

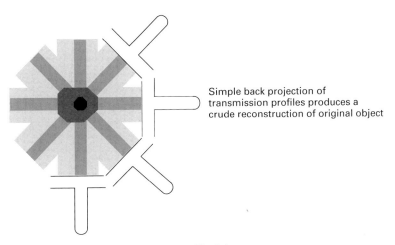

Simple back projection of
transmission profiles produces a
crude reconstruction of original object

Fig. 2.1

scanners used only a pencil beam of X-rays and a single detector which were moved in a translate–rotate manner around the patient. Subsequent innovations in hardware design have produced several generations of CT technology. Most scanners in current clinical use are third or fourth generation units with a collimated fan beam of X-rays and either an array of detectors mounted opposite to the X-ray tube, or a full ring of detectors completely surrounding the patient, which work sequentially as the fan beam rotates around the patient.

The patient is placed on a table which slides into the centre of the doughnut-shaped gantry housing. CT is essentially a tomographic technique giving images of slices of the patient's anatomy much as a loaf of bread may be sliced. Each slice may then be examined separately. In the CT scanner the slice location is determined by moving the patient in or out of the gantry housing. At a given slice location the gantry rotates around the patient with the transmitted radiation that passes through the patient measured by an array of many hundreds of detectors. In

the case of the machine we currently use, there are 768 detectors. The result is some 3 million measurements of transmitted radiation taken at multiple angles. From these measurements the computer makes calculations to fill in each square in a matrix 512 × 512 in size.

Pixels and voxels

Each square in this matrix is called a pixel or picture element. After the necessary calculations each pixel is assigned a digital value. This represents the X-ray absorption coefficient of all the tissue present within 1 voxel in the patient. A voxel is defined as the volume of tissue bounded by the dimensions of a pixel and the width of the X-ray beam. For example, in head scanning the machine is targeted so that the head fills the entire matrix (Fig. 2.2).

From this diagram it can be seen that each pixel is approximately 0.5 mm × 0.5 mm in dimensions. Pixel size is the limiting factor in spatial resolution in CT. For a standard head scan the best CT resolution currently

20 cm

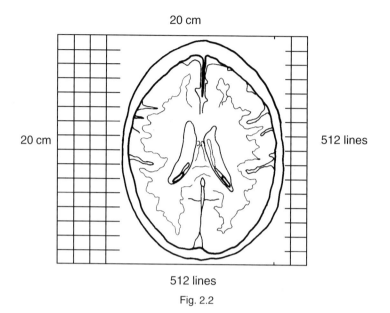

20 cm   512 lines

512 lines

Fig. 2.2

obtainable is of the order of 0.3–0.5 mm. This is less than is achievable on plain films, but is overshadowed immediately by the superior contrast resolution of CT which allows excellent tissue differentiation.

The width of the X-ray beam is usually 10 mm and hence each pixel value corresponds to the absorption coefficient of a volume or voxel of brain tissue measuring approximately 0.4 × 0.4 × 10 mm.

The width of the X-ray beam and thus the slice thickness is easily adjusted and most scanners give options of between 1–10 mm slice thickness.

Hounsfield units (Hu)

The digital value ascribed to each pixel is called the Hounsfield value (Fig. 2.3) which lies on a scale where pure water has a value 0 and air has a value of −1000. Bone has a value of the order of +1000.

The Hounsfield value reflects directly the

X-ray attenuation coefficient or electron density and thus the physical composition of the voxel of tissue that the pixel represents. The values for different tissue types are measurable and reproducible. Because they are recorded digitally they can be displayed, manipulated, interrogated and stored, thus giving an enormous range of diagnostic possibilities.

Most machines have a region of interest (ROI) capability which allows a small box on the machine monitor to be moved to an area of interest. The average Hounsfield value of all the pixels contained within that box is then displayed on the monitor. These pixel values are fundamental to the image and are not changed by any subsequent alterations in windowing or presentation (Fig. 2.4).

For easy visual interpretation each pixel is then ascribed a shade of grey, depending on its Hounsfield value and the windowing technique chosen (see below). Displayed in this form the electronic image is transferred

Positive

↑	+1000	Bone/Calcification
White	+70	Congealed blood
	+45	Grey matter
	+35	
	+30	White matter
Displayed on	+20	
spectrum of	+8	CSF
shades of grey		
(grey scale)	0	Reference point (pure water)
	−70	Fat
	−1000	Air
Black		
↓	Hounsfield Values, in Units (Hu)	
Negative	Not to scale	

Fig. 2.3

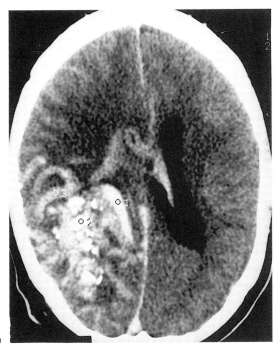

a

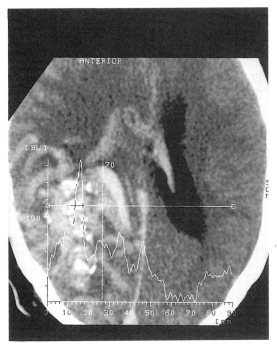

b

Fig. 2.4 a & b
(a) Contrast enhanced scan of large arteriovenous malformation. Three ROI readings differentiate between (1) congealed blood (78.6 Hu); (2) calcification (117.6 Hu) and (3) opacified blood within the malformation (58 Hu).
(b) A graphic representation of the same image showing a plot of absolute Hounsfield values across a single line of sight.

to hard copy film using a matrix or laser camera.

Windowing and grey scale

The average human eye can only differentiate some 30 shades of grey, despite the fact that most modern scan computers work with many more than this. The technique of windowing is an electronic manipulation of the data to enable these shades of grey to be used to represent a limited range, or window, of Hounsfield values. For standard cranial work the grey scale is compressed into a narrow window and distributed across only about 80 Hounsfield units. This means that with this setting the human eye can discriminate between tissues that are only 2 or 3 Hu apart in their attenuation. If several shades of grey intervene the eye separates them even more easily.

This is particularly important in cranial CT where grey and white matter, which are close to each other in Hounsfield values, must be discriminated.

At a compressed or narrow window of 80 Hu, centred on 30 Hu, everything with a Hounsfield value above 70 will appear white. It may be difficult to distinguish congealed blood reading 70 Hu from calcification reading 100 Hu or more. The absolute values or Hounsfield numbers do not however change and they can still be differentiated by taking individual readings of ROI at the console. Narrowing the window or compressing the grey scale thus increases contrast for the purposes of visual perception, without changing absolute values or disturbing relative radiographic tissue densities.

Conversely, widening the window will increase the range of Hounsfield numbers displayed in a single shade of grey. Spreading the window to span for example 1500 Hu with the 30 physiologically detectable shades of grey means that each shade encompasses 50 Hu. This means that most human soft tissue, and notably grey and white matter, will be displayed in the same shade of grey and will not be distinguishable from each other. Calcium or congealed blood would, however, be readily distinguishable from bone, a situation of clinical significance in the detection of an acute subdural haematoma or a calcified lesion adjacent to the cranial vault (Fig. 2.5). Critical CT scan findings could thus be obscured by inappropriate window settings. With the infinite possibility of display choices an unsuitable compromise for that particular clinical situation may have been selected.

Most cerebral scans are adequately viewed on a window setting of approximately 80 Hu units centred on 40 Hu. This is a good compromise which is serviceable for most clinical situations, as long as it is remembered that the computer stores a whole range of data which cannot be optimally shown on just one setting. If there is any doubt on the photographed images a quick resort to the console and to the region of interest facility will provide the absolute Hounsfield value information.

Most commonly, if important findings are missed on standard cranial CT displays, it is because wide (bone detail) windows have not been photographed to augment the routine series.

The preservation of relative tissue densities (Fig. 2.3), regardless of the windowing technique used, is a valuable concept in CT which is lost in the allied modality of MRI. In CT, unless the image is photographically inverted, bone will always be denser than soft tissue which will in turn exceed that of fat

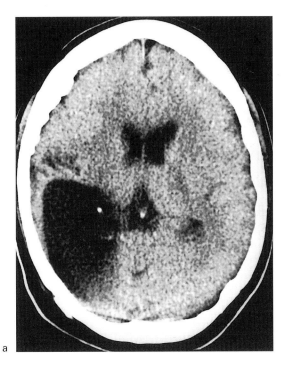 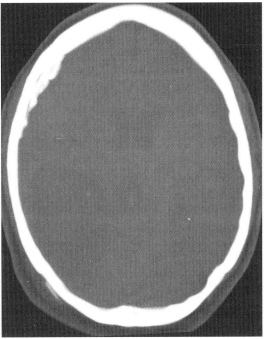

a

b

Fig. 2.5 a & b
(a) A narrow window setting (W66, C38) displays the calcified chronic right frontal subdural haematoma as white, and indistinguishable from the adjacent skull. There is incidental porencephalic dilatation of the R trigone.
(b) A wide setting (W2126, C552) of the same slice clearly distinguishes the calcium from the bone, but with complete loss of contrast among the intracranial tissues.

and air. Independent of the window, it is thus usually possible to assess the physical composition of a lesion by comparing it with the density of readily identifiable anatomic structures on the same slice such as the ventricles with their CSF, the scalp with its fat and the paranasal sinuses with their air.

Partial volume and 3-dimensionality

The Hounsfield number, and hence the shade of grey ascribed to any single voxel, will reflect the average density of the tissue it contains. A small component of very high density material 'contaminating' the voxel will thus result in the whole pixel being ascribed a higher Hounsfield number. The thicker the slice the more likely this is to happen (Fig. 2.6a).

This occurs frequently in cranial CT, involving the clinoid processes, the jugular tubercles, the arcuate eminence of the sphenoid and bony irregularities found in the axial plane, such as those along the floor of the anterior cranial fossa.

Similarly if low density CSF or fat is partially included on the slice then all voxels containing such material will appear lower in density.

Review of the slices immediately above and below the slice in question will demonstrate the cause of any partial volume effect by showing the 3-dimensional nature of a

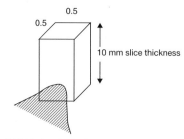

(a) Bone (high H.u.) projecting into voxel is averaged with surrounding soft tissue (lower H.u.)

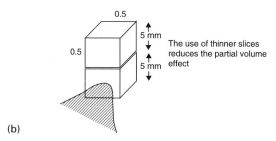

(b)

Fig. 2.6 a & b

structure. Adjacent slices will also confirm the shape of a structure or lesion which may be round, tubular or wedge-shaped. These will have a major impact on interpretation.

Partial volume is not a true artefact but an inevitable consequence of the finite slice thickness. A thinner slice will reduce the partial volume effect (Fig. 2.6b).

iii. Technique

Generation of the scout image

There are many possible variations, depending on the desired field of coverage, the nature of the tissue suspected to be abnormal, and the constraints imposed by the anatomy and radiation dose. The patient usually lies supine on the scanning couch and is advanced towards the scanning field in the gantry. A scout image is generated by energizing the X-ray beam and passing the relevant part of the patient in one movement through the gantry. This continuous exposure as the patient moves through the beam generates a topogram which resembles a plain X-ray. In the case of the head, this is usually a lateral image of the skull though frontal projections are also possible. It is by nature a digital image and thus the windowing options already described can also be applied to it.

From this scout image the position, number and angulation of the subsequent slices are chosen.

Choice of imaging plane

Axial

The axial plane is the one most readily available on CT and can easily be obtained in most supine patients.

Occasionally an obtunded patient will not

maintain a supine position, or there may be reasons for the patient to be nursed in the decubitus position. Providing adequate immobilization is ensured there is no reason why adequate axial images cannot be obtained in this position.

The axial plane offers the advantage of direct left–right comparison, which is useful in a symmetrical structure like the head. There are a few caveats, notably related to the curved shape of the head (Fig. 2.7).

Coronal

This is another very useful plane. It also allows left–right comparisons and has the geometric advantage of offering scans at right angles to major bony structures such as the floors of the anterior and middle cranial fossac, the orbital roof and floor and the hard palate.

Orthogonal or right-angled imaging is extremely useful. Its value is emphasized wherever a number of tissue layers are closely spaced in the same plane, and where that plane has the same orientation as the prescribed slice. For example, the cortex of the frontal lobes lies in the axial plane as does the layer of CSF between it and the floor of the anterior cranial fossa. Trying to assess these structures with axial slices, especially where the thickness of the structure may be less than the slice thickness, can lead to

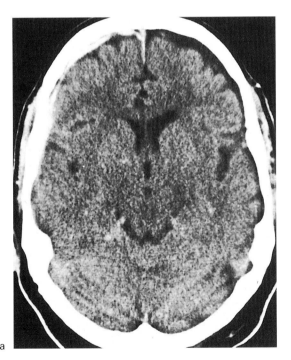
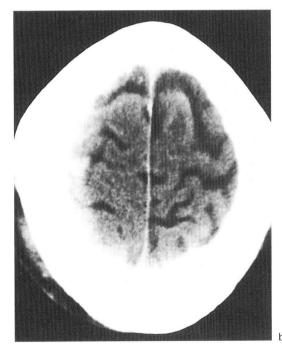

a

b

Fig. 2.7 a & b
The influence of cranial curvature on the shape of pathology.
(a) Shallow fresh R subdural haematoma which is hyperdense with respect to adjacent brain. In the mid-cranium the X-ray beam intersects the skull and the collection almost perpendicularly, producing clean, sharp margins.
(b) At the vertex, in the same patient, the beam intersects the haematoma tangentially as it curves up and over the brain surface. It appears larger than it did inferiorly, because the beam is coursing through the long rather than the short axis of the collection. The margin appears less distinct.

significant partial volume averaging problems.

Coronal scans will clarify the relationship of a lesion to all structures running in a roughly axial plane, including the tentorium cerebelli which on its medial aspect is angled superiorly but elsewhere has a more-or-less axial orientation (Fig. 2.8). Knowledge of the compartmental localization of pathology is fundamental in guiding a neurosurgical approach.

The best coronal images are obtained directly, with the patient prone with the neck in hyperextension, or supine in a 'hanging head' position. This may not be feasible in injured patients or those with cervical spondylosis or vertebrobasilar insufficiency.

Computer-generated reformations then provide a crude but reasonable alternative. They cannot by definition add new real digital information, and in fact usually appear somewhat primitive and 'blocky'. They can, however, add an additional display or dimension from existing data. This may help the analysis of the image, and display it in an orientation to which the clinician can relate.

Sagittal

Sagittal images are splendid for midline unpaired structures such as the corpus callosum, pineal, pituitary, aqueduct and spinal cord, as MRI has confirmed, and also, like coronal scans, for transcranial pathology. Unfortunately, due to anatomic constraints,

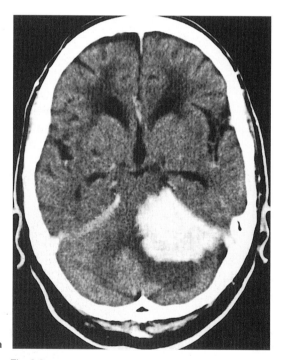
a

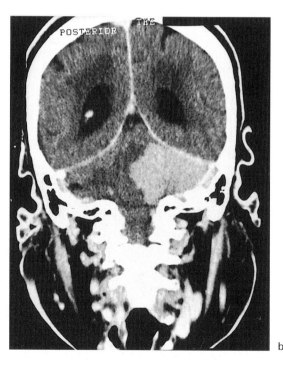
b

Fig. 2.8
(a) Contrast enhanced scan (+C) of meningioma. Because the scan is angled parallel to the skull base, the frontal horns of the lateral ventricles and this posterior fossa tumour are shown on the same slice.
(b) Direct coronal scan in the same patient shows the true 3-dimensional arrangement within the head, and confirms the sessile semilunar shape of the tumour and its relationship to the superiorly angled leaf of the tentorium.

direct sagittal scans are almost impossible in cranial CT, and one has to rely on reformations (Fig. 2.9). Contiguous slices (with no inter-slice gaps) are required and a slight degree of overlap helps smooth the reformatted image. Finer slices also improve image quality by reducing the 'blockiness', but at the cost of radiation dose.

Other projections and implications

Other variations on these classical planes may be used. For example, an off-coronal orientation may be chosen to avoid high density dental amalgam or other metal which would produce streak artefacts across the slice.

Other patient positions can exploit the effects of gravity. True air–fluid or fluid–fluid levels can be confirmed by tilting the patient's head slightly and repositioning the apparent level. This may confirm the presence of small quantities of blood or heavy particulate matter in the dependent portions of the ventricles, and distinguish these from partial volume averaging artefacts. Collections of air may also be moved around within the head, as in the use of the decubitus position to move introduced subarachnoid air to outline a cerebellopontine angle tumour.

The supine position may also cause a shrunken brain to drop back within the skull, creating a false impression of selective frontal atrophy.

Slice thickness

Almost as much radiation is used to produce any slice regardless of its thickness. If the whole head were scanned with 1 mm rather than 10 mm slices, ten times the radiation dose would be given and it would take ten

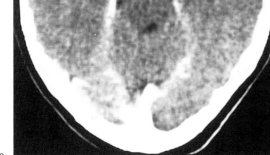

a

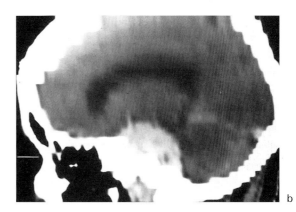

b

Fig. 2.9 a & b
(a) Axial scan (+C) showing intensely enhancing chemodectoma. Its true anatomic extent cannot be appreciated on this single slice.
(b) Computer generated sagittal reformation which appears somewhat crude but which shows the shape of the tumour and its transcranial extension.

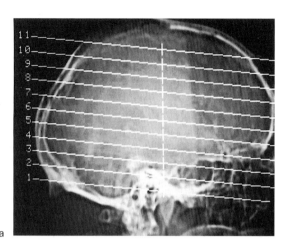

a

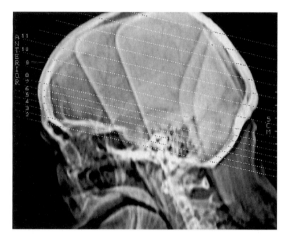

b

Fig. 2.10a
Scout film with traditional/standard slices prescribed.
There are contiguous 10 mm slices parallel to the
infraorbito-meatal line. Note the large myelomatous lytic
lesions at the vertex and in the outer table of the frontal
bone. The lesion at the vertex could be missed. The scout
should be checked in case the protocol needs adaptation
to the clinical situation.

Fig. 2.10b
Angled axial scan with finer basal slices.

times longer. If however, one were confined
to 10 mm axial slices, the maximal resolution
in the vertical plane would be restricted to
10 mm. If the suspected pathology is
significantly smaller than this, or if finer
detail is required, then it is appropriate to
use thinner slices. For example, the pituitary
fossa can be imaged on one single 10 mm
thick slice which will give little detailed information as to abnormalities within the fossa.
One or 2 mm thick slices significantly improve
image information. Thinner slices (usually
5 mm in thickness) are also commonly used
in the posterior fossa to improve resolution
and to reduce the beam hardening artefacts
which occur here.

Number and position of slices

Once the slice thickness and angulation have
been decided, the number of slices and their
location are chosen on the basis of the number of scans required to cover the area of
clinical interest. Standard protocols are a
compromise between image detail and cost
benefit, including wear and tear to the equip-
ment in the form of tube heating and also
radiation dose to the patient.

Standard protocols

Standard traditional head scan
Thick contiguous axial slices are performed
parallel to one of the commonly used radiographic baselines, such as the infraorbito-
meatal line. Depending on the manufacturing
design, such slices are usually 8 or 10 mm
thick. This is the simplest protocol and was
widely used in the early years of CT operation (Fig. 2.10a).

Posterior fossa/angled axial scan
Here the scan is angled at 20° to the baseline
or, more simply, parallel to the skull base. An
added refinement is the use of finer (5 mm)
slices inferiorly through the posterior fossa,
reverting to standard 10 mm slices at the
level of the tentorium (Fig. 2.10b).

This protocol is now widely used.

Scanning with this angulation to the standard baseline introduces some distortion into the traditional appearance of the intracranial contents. The lateral ventricles are no longer routinely sliced along their longest axes, and appear foreshortened, and the brainstem appears smaller. One quickly adapts to such changes, however, and the benefits in terms of improved image quality and ease of examination performance easily outweigh the disadvantages. Detail in the posterior fossa is improved with this technique and the scan no longer includes the orbits, thus reducing the dose to the radiation-sensitive lens of the eye.

Middle cranial fossa

A reverse posterior fossa angulation can be used to reduce the beam hardening artefact across the temporal lobes due to the irregular bony surface of the middle cranial fossa. Enthusiasm for this technique has waned with the acknowledgement of the value of magnetic resonance in this area.

Inner or middle ear scans

1 or 2 mm thick slices at 30° to the standard baseline with or without coronals (i.e. 100° to baseline).

Pituitary

1 or 2 mm thick coronal slices.

Intravenous contrast – to use or not to use

Until the contrast syringe is grasped a CT head scan is a non-invasive safe procedure. The injection of intravenous contrast, even of the non-ionic variety, adds a small but nonetheless significant risk (of the order of 1 in 40 000) of allergic reaction and patient death. There are also minor reactions such as vomiting, which are quite common with the use of ionic agents. Though not life-threatening, these hinder the performance of the scan and distress the patient.

In the early days of scanning when images were crude, intravenous contrast was used routinely to opacify useful landmarks such as the circle of Willis. With improved image quality this is seldom necessary, and many head scans are now performed unenhanced. Contrast agents should be injected on a rational basis with a clear understanding of how they will improve the diagnostic efficacy of any individual examination.

Intravenous contrast contains iodine which is of high density and increases the local absorption coefficient, making the area appear whiter on the scan.

When a contrast agent is injected intravenously it is initially almost entirely contained within the vascular space. If scans are performed early both normal and abnormal vessels appear markedly enhanced. Normal cerebral tissue does not enhance, because of the presence of a blood–brain barrier (BBB) which maintains the homeostasis of the neuronal environment.

This barrier is formed by the presence of tight capillary junctions. The functional result is that the endothelium of cerebral capillaries acts as a semipermeable membrane preventing the passage of large molecules such as contrast ions into the extravascular space. If the BBB is damaged or poorly developed, contrast leaks into the extravascular space. This principle underlies contrast enhancement in many intra-axial tumours and inflammatory processes. It takes some minutes for this leakage to occur and thus the post contrast scan should not be hurried. In fact large dose delayed scans up to 1 hour after injection used to be the preferred method of detecting actively demyelinating plaques or metastases prior to the advent of MR.

Normal extra-axial structures such as the anterior pituitary gland lack a BBB and enhance routinely. Extra-axial lesions such as meningiomas and Schwannomas enhance strongly for the same reason, complementing their intrinsic vascularity.

The injection of contrast thus has two roles:

1. To enable detection of a lesion.
   Rarely is a clinically significant lesion not detectable on plain scans due to mass effect or density variation, but intravenous contrast is needed for notoriously occult or isodense lesions without significant mass effect. These include some cerebellopontine angle tumours and small vascular malformations. The absolute yield of detected lesions may also increase, and, for example, confirm that neoplasia is metastatic rather than primary.
2. To enable characterization of a lesion.
   Once a lesion is detected on a plain scan the injection of contrast narrows the differential diagnosis (DD) by providing more information about the macropathology or physical nature of the lesion.

Rates and patterns of contrast enhancement will be discussed further in Chapter 5.

As a broad generalization, intravenous contrast is usually not used in the investigation of conditions with global dysfunction without focal signs. Such conditions include dementia, headache, and psychiatric illness. It is seldom used in acute clinical cere-

brovascular accidents or recent trauma or haemorrhage. In these conditions it adds little useful diagnostic information, and may obscure important findings such as sub-arachnoid haemorrhage.

It is generally administered routinely in the investigation of:

– pituitary abnormality
– suspected cerebellopontine (CP) angle tumour
– first investigation of focal seizure
– recent onset of focal neurological signs or symptoms

or if an abnormality is demonstrated on plain scans which requires further characterization.

In most cases a standard manual injection of 50 cc of an agent with an iodine content of over 300 mg/ml will be sufficient. Rarely is there a need for larger doses or more sophisticated administration protocols in cranial scanning, though dynamic and spiral techniques are giving increasingly accurate and complex demonstration of major vessel anatomy and pathology.

At all times the implications of increasing the patient risk, the radiation exposure, the complexity of the procedure and its cost should be balanced against the implications for the management of the individual patient.

Artefacts

The image may be degraded by artefacts resulting from machinery malfunction, patient movement, or structures present within the slice being scanned.

Technical artefacts
A whole range of technical malfunctions are possible in a CT scanner most of which

result in complete failure of image production. However, ring artefacts caused by single detector malfunctions allow the production of a degraded image. The rings are usually located centrally within the scan and are repeated on a number of slices. Not all scanners are susceptible to this artefact.

Patient motion artefact

If all the structures contained within a slice do not remain motionless throughout the scan time a degraded image results. Thankfully, head scanning is not susceptible to breathing or cardiac motion artefact but patients having head scans may by nature of their illness be relatively non-cooperative. The shortening of scan times with improved technology has thus improved image quality and also improved patient safety by reducing the need for sedation.

Artefacts due to structures contained within the slice

- *Beam hardening artefact*

All X-ray tubes are like light bulbs and produce a spectrum of radiation. The X-ray tube in a CT scanner thus emits radiation of varying energy. The greater the energy the less it is absorbed and the reverse is true for lower energy radiation. As an X-ray beam passes through bone all the lower energies are absorbed. The resultant emerging beam has a higher average energy and is said to be hardened. If it then passes through brain less of the beam will be absorbed than if it had not first been filtered by bone.

It is difficult for the scan computer to deal with this beam hardening effect, especially when the beam passes through a lot of bone and not much brain, as in the posterior fossa. The result is a streak artefact across the brain tissue. This so-called interpetrous artefact ultimately limits the usefulness of CT in the

posterior fossa. It is characterized by a linear band of low attenuation connecting two areas of high density such as bone. The tissue traversed by this artefact is displayed with degraded information. Similar problems are seen in the middle cranial fossa.

- *Metal artefact*

The X-ray absorption coefficient of metal is much higher than any other structure found in the human body. Even a small amount of metal in a single slice will result in quite a dramatic streak artefact extending across the remainder of the image. In head scans this is encountered with surgical clips, gunshot debris, dental amalgam or other extraneous objects (Fig. 2.11).

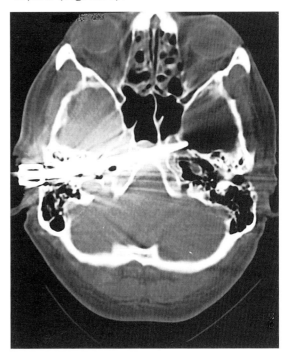

Fig. 2.11
Plain scan, W672. Suicide attempt by insertion of screwdriver into R ear. At narrower window settings the metallic artefact was so severe the image was difficult to interpret. Widening the window has reduced intracranial detail but also the metallic artefact, and clarified the relationship between the foreign body and the skull base.

Bibliography

Burman S, Rosenbaum A E 1982 Rationale and techniques for intravenous enhancement in computed tomography. Radiologic Clinics of North America 20(1): 15–22

Gedroyc W, Rankin S 1992 Practical CT techniques. Springer, London

Hendee W R 1983 The physical principles of computed tomography. Little, Brown, Boston

Lange S, Grumme T, Kluge W, Ringel K, Meese W 1989 Cerebral and spinal computerised tomography. Schering, Berlin

Sage M R 1982 Blood–brain barrier: phenomenon of increasing importance to the imaging clinician. American Journal of Neuroradiology 3: 127–138

CHAPTER 3

Normal anatomy

Eight representative axial CT slices are presented, taken parallel to the skull base and ascending sequentially to the vertex. The slices are displayed as if viewed from the feet. Matching line diagrams accompany them, listing the major points of interest. Additional diagrams supply further detail for the purposes of clinico-pathological correlation.

The anatomy is then approached in terms of the vascular territories of the brain.

Slice 1

This slice (Fig. 3.1) passes through the inferior posterior fossa and middle cranial fossa. This slice unavoidably passes through a large amount of dense bone in the petrous ridges and sphenoid wings and the resultant streak artefact limits visualization of normal anatomy. Finer slices will reduce this artefact if necessary.

The slice passes through the medulla and although CT imaging of this region is limited a basic diagram of the normal anatomy of the medulla is included (Fig. 3.2).

The sella turcica is included on this scan but for the pituitary gland direct coronal views are recommended. The normal anatomy of this region has been illustrated separately (Fig. 3.3).

The petrous bones are included too but specific abnormalities of these structures require finer slices (Fig. 3.4).

A series of fine slices through the base of skull displayed on bone windows is included to demonstrate the important foramina within it (Fig. 3.5). The accompanying table lists the structures passing through these foramina (Table 3.1).

Table 3.1
Structures passing through cranial foramina

Foramen rotundum
Maxillary nerve V2 into pterygopalatine fossa

Foramen ovale
Mandibular nerve V3
Accessory meningeal artery

Foramen spinosum
Middle meningeal artery and vein
Meningeal branches of mandibular nerve

Internal auditory meatus
Facial VII nerve
Vestibulo-cochlear VIII nerve
Inferior auditory artery

Stylomastoid foramen
Facial nerve

Foramen lacerum
Carotid canal
Internal carotid artery
Sympathetic nerve

Jugular foramen
Anteromedial part
Inferior petrosal sinus
Meningeal branch of ascending pharyngeal artery
Middle part – Glossopharyngeal IX, Vagus X,
Accessory XI cranial nerves
Posterolateral part
Jugular vein
Meningeal branches of occipital artery and of vagus
nerve

Hypoglossal canal
Hypoglossal XII nerve

Pterygoid canal
Vidian artery

Superior orbital fissure
Oculomotor III nerve
Trochlear IV nerve
Abducent VI nerve
Ophthalmic division of trigeminal V1 nerve
Superior Ophthalmic vein

Optic foramen
Optic nerve II
Ophthalmic artery

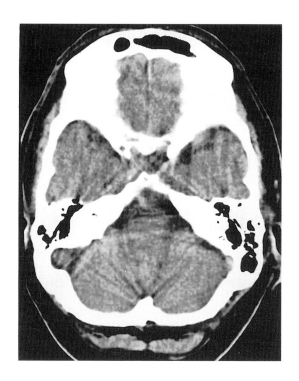

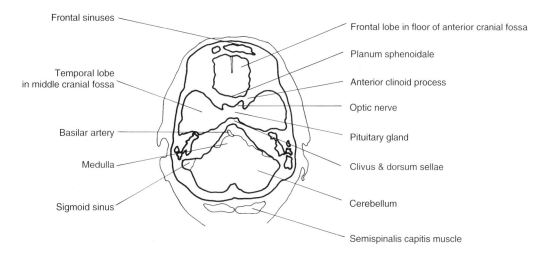

Frontal sinuses

Frontal lobe in floor of anterior cranial fossa

Planum sphenoidale

Temporal lobe
in middle cranial fossa

Anterior clinoid process

Optic nerve

Basilar artery

Pituitary gland

Medulla

Clivus & dorsum sellae

Sigmoid sinus

Cerebellum

Semispinalis capitis muscle

Fig. 3.1
Slice 1.

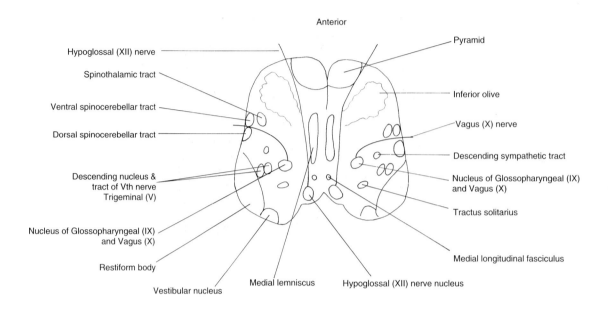

Fig. 3.2
Axial anatomy of medulla.

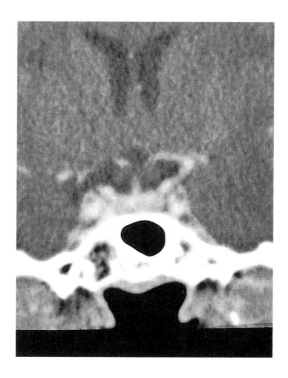

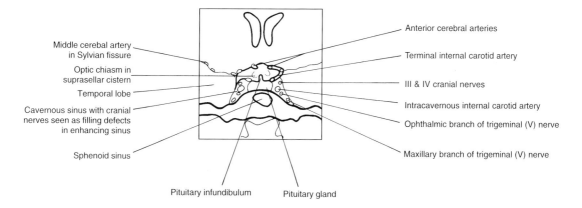

Middle cerebal artery in Sylvian fissure

Optic chiasm in suprasellar cistern

Temporal lobe

Cavernous sinus with cranial nerves seen as filling defects in enhancing sinus

Sphenoid sinus

Pituitary infundibulum

Pituitary gland

Anterior cerebral arteries

Terminal internal carotid artery

III & IV cranial nerves

Intracavernous internal carotid artery

Ophthalmic branch of trigeminal (V) nerve

Maxillary branch of trigeminal (V) nerve

Fig. 3.3
Coronal anatomy of pituitary.

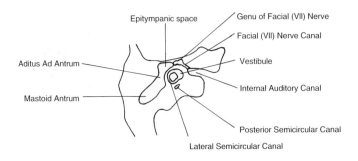

Epitympanic space — Genu of Facial (VII) Nerve
Facial (VII) Nerve Canal
Aditus Ad Antrum — Vestibule
Mastoid Antrum — Internal Auditory Canal
Posterior Semicircular Canal
Lateral Semicircular Canal

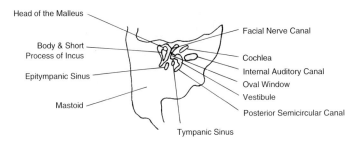

Head of the Malleus — Facial Nerve Canal
Body & Short Process of Incus — Cochlea
Epitympanic Sinus — Internal Auditory Canal
Oval Window
Mastoid — Vestibule
Posterior Semicircular Canal
Tympanic Sinus

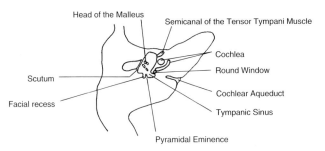

Head of the Malleus — Semicanal of the Tensor Tympani Muscle
Cochlea
Round Window
Scutum — Cochlear Aqueduct
Facial recess — Tympanic Sinus
Pyramidal Eminence

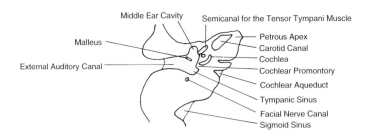

Middle Ear Cavity — Semicanal for the Tensor Tympani Muscle
Petrous Apex
Malleus — Carotid Canal
Cochlea
External Auditory Canal — Cochlear Promontory
Cochlear Aqueduct
Tympanic Sinus
Facial Nerve Canal
Sigmoid Sinus

Fig. 3.4a
Axial images of R petrous bone from superior to inferior.

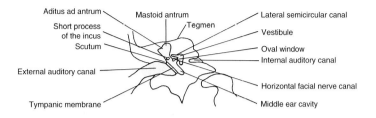

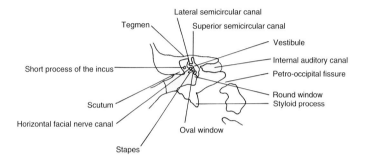

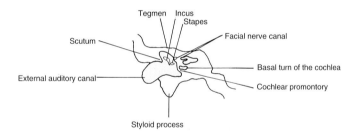

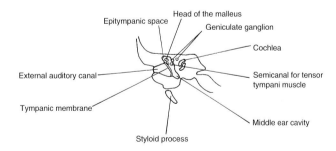

Fig. 3.4b
Coronal images of R petrous bone from posterior to anterior.

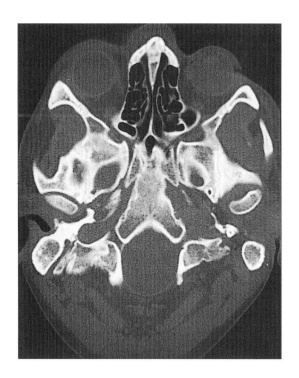

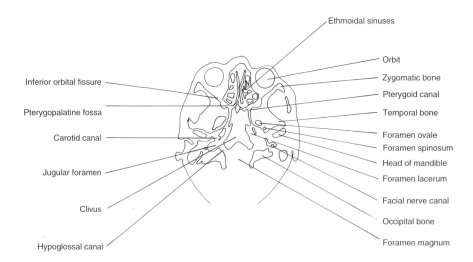

Fig. 3.5 (1)
Base of skull.

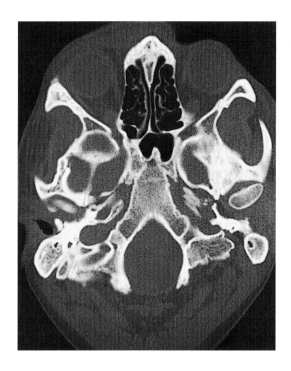

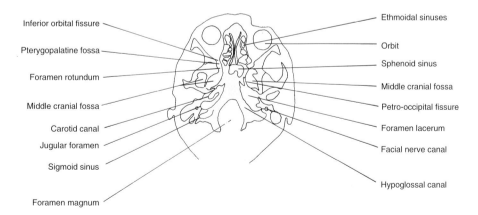

Inferior orbital fissure

Pterygopalatine fossa

Foramen rotundum

Middle cranial fossa

Carotid canal

Jugular foramen

Sigmoid sinus

Foramen magnum

Ethmoidal sinuses

Orbit

Sphenoid sinus

Middle cranial fossa

Petro-occipital fissure

Foramen lacerum

Facial nerve canal

Hypoglossal canal

Fig. 3.5 (2)
Base of skull.

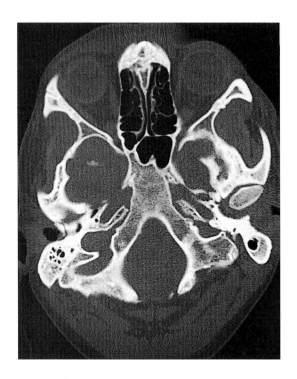

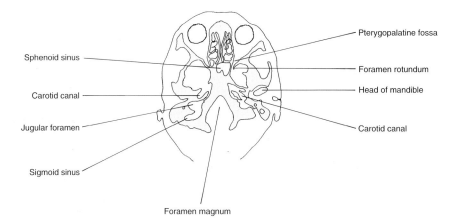

Fig. 3.5 (3)
Base of skull.

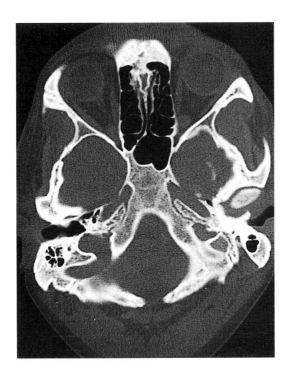

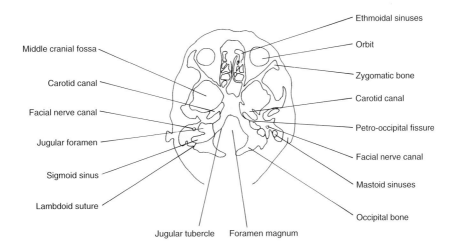

Fig. 3.5 (4)
Base of skull.

Slice 2

This slice passes more superiorly through the posterior fossa (Fig. 3.6). The pons is included on this scan and basic pontine anatomy is shown in the accompanying diagram (Fig. 3.7). The pons forms the floor of the fourth ventricle (V4) which should be seen centrally in the posterior fossa on this slice. The cerebellum forms an integral part of the extrapyramidal system and has an essential role in the co-ordination of group muscle activities. The cerebellum is connected to the brain stem by three cerebellar peduncles. The inferior, middle and superior cerebellar peduncles connect the medulla, pons and midbrain respectively, and on this image the middle cerebellar peduncle is seen, connecting the cerebellum to the pons.

The cerebellum is divided into two large hemispheres with a narrow median vermis. The nodulus of the posterior vermis and the attached flocculi form the flocculonodular lobe. The flocculi lie close to the cerebello-pontine angle and can be misinterpreted as an abnormal mass in this region. The anterolateral limits of the choroid plexus of V4 can protrude adjacent to the flocculus and may be mistaken for a small enhancing mass.

The basilar artery lies immediately anterior to the pons and in older patients can be quite tortuous, deviating towards the cerebellopontine angles.

The dorsum sellae and anterior clinoid processes may be only partially included on the slice, resulting in a partial volume effect where they mimic internal carotid artery aneurysms.

The temporal lobe fills the middle cranial fossa. With scans angled parallel to the skull base the tips of the temporal horns of the lateral ventricles are customarily visualized in normal patients.

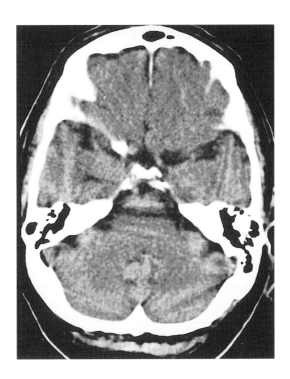

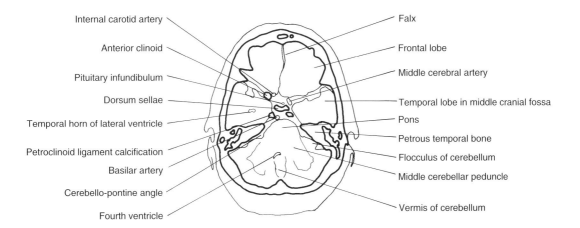

Internal carotid artery

Anterior clinoid

Pituitary infundibulum

Dorsum sellae

Temporal horn of lateral ventricle

Petroclinoid ligament calcification

Basilar artery

Cerebello-pontine angle

Fourth ventricle

Falx

Frontal lobe

Middle cerebral artery

Temporal lobe in middle cranial fossa

Pons

Petrous temporal bone

Flocculus of cerebellum

Middle cerebellar peduncle

Vermis of cerebellum

Fig. 3.6
Slice 2.

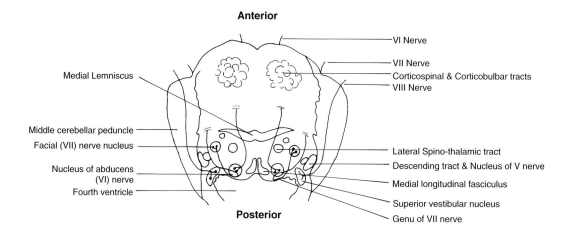

Fig. 3.7
Pons.

Slice 3

This slice (Fig. 3.8) passes more superiorly through the pons and posterior fossa. The fourth ventricle is well seen as a midline structure within the posterior fossa. The nodulus of the cerebellum indents the posterior aspect of V4.

The suprasellar cistern lies anterior to the pons and within this region segments of the circle of Willis are usually evident. The normal configuration of the circle of Willis is demonstrated in the accompanying diagram (Fig. 3.9). Berry aneurysms commonly arise from the anterior communicating artery (A), from the origin of the posterior communicating artery (B), from the bifurcation of the middle cerebral artery (C) and the apex of the basilar artery (D). The first three sites each account for approximately 30% of berry aneurysms whilst the basilar tip accounts for some 10%. Origins from other vessels are rare, with the posterior inferior cerebellar artery being most important. These sites warrant specific attention on this slice. The lateral view of the arteries of the brain is also included for reference (Fig. 3.10). Arterial territories within the brain are discussed separately.

The superior tips of the clinoid processes are visible and the pituitary infundibulum is variably identified centrally within the pituitary fossa. The temporal lobe in the middle cranial fossa is seen lateral to the suprasellar cistern and the temporal horns are visible centrally. Anteriorly, the frontal lobes occupy the anterior cranial fossa.

Normal anatomy

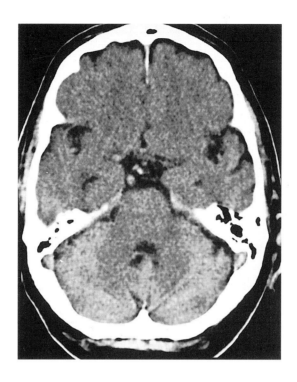

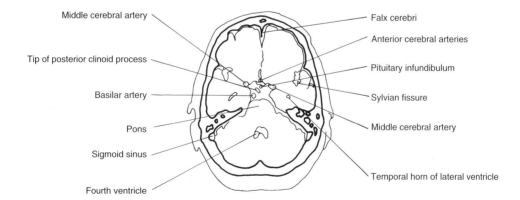

Middle cerebral artery

Tip of posterior clinoid process

Basilar artery

Pons

Sigmoid sinus

Fourth ventricle

Falx cerebri

Anterior cerebral arteries

Pituitary infundibulum

Sylvian fissure

Middle cerebral artery

Temporal horn of lateral ventricle

Fig. 3.8
Slice 3.

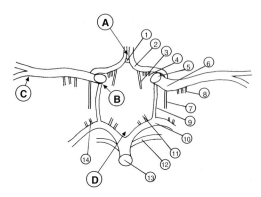

1. Anterior communicating artery
2. Anterior cerebral artery
3. Recurrent artery of Heubner
4. Antero medial perforating arteries
5. Terminal internal artery carotid artery
6. Middle cerebral artery
7. Anterior choroidal artery
8. Lenticulostriate arteries
9. Posterior communicating artery
10. Posterior cerebral artery
11. Thalamo perforating vessels
12. Superior cerebellar artery
13. Basilar artery
14. Postero lateral choroidal arteries

Fig. 3.9
Circle of Willis.

Normal anatomy

(LATERAL VIEW)

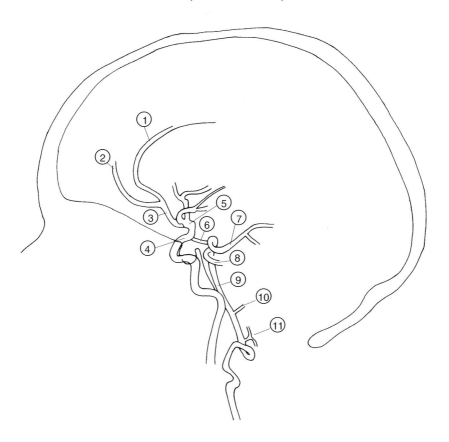

① Pericallosal
② Calloso marginal
③ Anterior cerebral

④ Internal carotid artery
⑤ Middle cerebral artery
    and branches
⑥ Posterior Communicating artery
⑦ Posterior cerebral artery
⑧ Superior cerebellar artery

⑨ Basilar artery
⑩ Anterior inferior cerebellar artery
⑪ Posterior inferior cerebellar artery

Fig. 3.10
Arteries of the brain (lateral view).

Slice 4

This slice (Fig. 3.11) passes through the midbrain and superior cerebellum. The supero-lateral margins of the cerebellum are demarcated by the tentorium cerebelli which divides the posterior fossa from the occipital lobes. As the tentorium passes obliquely through the scan plane it is usually not clearly defined but its location can be deduced. This area should be specifically assessed for extracerebral haemorrhage which may collect over the tentorium.

The midbrain is the short portion of the brain between the pons and cerebral hemispheres. The dorsal portion of the midbrain (the tectum) contains the four corpora quadrigemina while the ventrolateral portions contain the two cerebral peduncles. The corpora quadrigemina consist of the four rounded eminences of the superior and inferior colliculi. The colliculi have a role in eye movement and lesions in this region and the nearby pineal can produce paralysis of upward gaze (Parinaud's syndrome). The midbrain also contains the red nuclei and substantia nigra (Fig. 3.12). Both of these structures are involved in the extrapyramidal system and lesions here may produce a Parkinsonian picture.

The CSF space posterior to the colliculi is commonly referred to as the quadrigeminal plate cistern. This connects around the midbrain via the ambient cistern with the pre-pontine cistern anteriorly. The cerebral aqueduct of Sylvius passing posteriorly through the midbrain is usually too small to be defined on CT but this area should be specifically examined if there is evidence of hydrocephalus involving only the third and lateral ventricles.

The lower limits of the third ventricle are seen on this slice and immediately posterior and inferior to this are the paired mammillary nuclei of the hypothalamus which may atrophy in alcoholism.

The Sylvian fissures seen laterally delineate the frontal lobe from the temporal lobe and contain branches of the middle cerebral artery. The anterior lip of the Sylvian fissure is the operculum of the inferior frontal gyrus which contains the motor area of language (Broca's area). Language areas are lateralized in one hemisphere and, in at least 95% of all individuals, especially those who are right-handed, this is the left hemisphere. In left-handed persons a dominance of the left hemisphere is present in about 60%. The sensory area of language (Wernicke's area) lies in the superior temporal gyrus between the primary auditory cortex and the angular gyrus and is seen on more superior scans (5 and 6). An expressive aphasia is usually due to a lesion in Broca's area and a receptive aphasia due to a lesion in Wernicke's area.

Normal anatomy

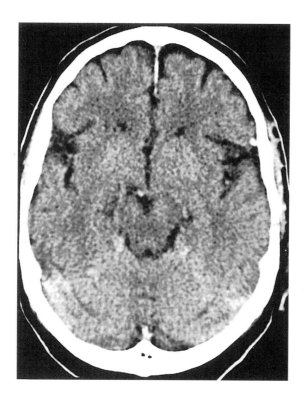

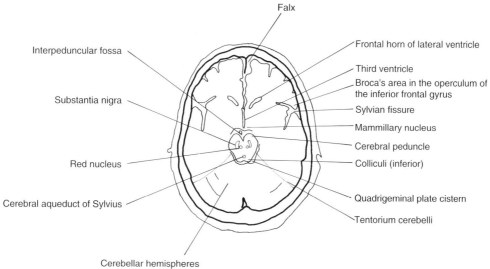

Falx

Interpeduncular fossa

Frontal horn of lateral ventricle

Third ventricle

Broca's area in the operculum of
the inferior frontal gyrus

Sylvian fissure

Substantia nigra

Mammillary nucleus

Cerebral peduncle

Red nucleus

Colliculi (inferior)

Quadrigeminal plate cistern

Cerebral aqueduct of Sylvius

Tentorium cerebelli

Cerebellar hemispheres

Fig. 3.11
Slice 4.

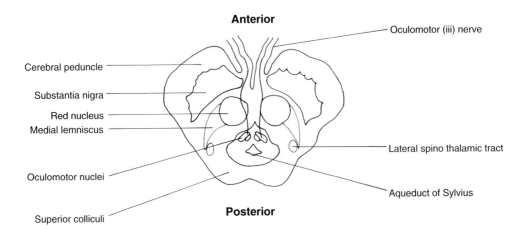

Anterior

Oculomotor (iii) nerve

Cerebral peduncle

Substantia nigra

Red nucleus

Medial lemniscus

Lateral spino thalamic tract

Oculomotor nuclei

Aqueduct of Sylvius

Superior colliculi

Posterior

Fig. 3.12
Midbrain.

Slice 5

This slice (Fig. 3.13) passes through the middle of the third ventricle and includes the thalami and internal capsules. This area is highlighted in the accompanying diagram (Fig. 3.14). The anterior limb of the internal capsule is usually supplied by the recurrent artery of Heubner. An infarct in this territory usually produces a mild aphasia and some extrapyramidal rigidity. The posterior limb of the internal capsule is supplied by the anterior choroidal artery and an infarct here produces a dense hemiplegia, an incomplete hemianaesthesia and an upper quadrant hemianopia.

The third ventricle (V3) is seen centrally and is connected anteriorly with the two frontal horns of the lateral ventricles by the foramina of Monro. Hydrocephalus limited to the lateral ventricles should require specific examination of this region for exclusion of a colloid cyst. V3 is bounded posteriorly by the habenular commissure, pineal gland and posterior commissure from superior to inferior. The pineal gland is calcified in virtually all adult CT head scans and also in a high percentage of children. Pineal gland calcification over 1 cm in diameter should be regarded with suspicion.

The Sylvian fissures are again seen laterally overlying the insula. The extreme capsule, claustrum and external capsule all lie within the insula. The external capsule defines the outer limits of the lentiform nucleus which consists of the putamen and globus pallidus. These structures, along with the caudate nucleus, amygdaloid body and claustrum, represent the basal ganglia.

More posteriorly, the upper margin of the tentorium cerebelli is visible with a small portion of the vermis of the cerebellum seen protruding through the tentorial hiatus. The quadrigeminal plate cistern is once again seen along the posterior aspect of the superior colliculi.

The ventricular and cisternal configuration on this slice is reminiscent of a smiling face, with the frontal horns as eyes, V3 as the nose and the quadrigeminal plate cistern as the mouth. Disturbances to this recognizable pattern require an explanation, with deformity or flattening of the grin, for example, being an early sign of a subtle space-occupying process in the brainstem or superior cerebellum.

Normal anatomy

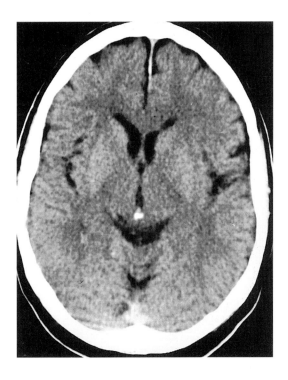

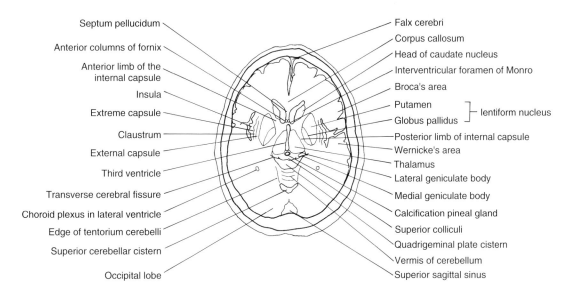

Septum pellucidum

Anterior columns of fornix

Anterior limb of the
internal capsule

Insula

Extreme capsule

Claustrum

External capsule

Third ventricle

Transverse cerebral fissure

Choroid plexus in lateral ventricle

Edge of tentorium cerebelli

Superior cerebellar cistern

Occipital lobe

Falx cerebri

Corpus callosum

Head of caudate nucleus

Interventricular foramen of Monro

Broca's area

Putamen

Globus pallidus — lentiform nucleus

Posterior limb of internal capsule

Wernicke's area

Thalamus

Lateral geniculate body

Medial geniculate body

Calcification pineal gland

Superior colliculi

Quadrigeminal plate cistern

Vermis of cerebellum

Superior sagittal sinus

Fig. 3.13
Slice 5.

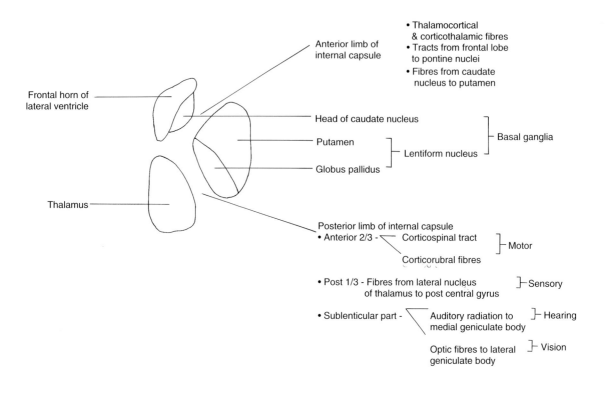

Anterior limb of internal capsule
- Thalamocortical & corticothalamic fibres
- Tracts from frontal lobe to pontine nuclei
- Fibres from caudate nucleus to putamen

Frontal horn of lateral ventricle

Head of caudate nucleus

Putamen ⎤
Globus pallidus ⎦ Lentiform nucleus ⎤ Basal ganglia

Thalamus

Posterior limb of internal capsule
- Anterior 2/3 - Corticospinal tract ⎤ Motor
  Corticorubral fibres ⎦

- Post 1/3 - Fibres from lateral nucleus of thalamus to post central gyrus ⎤ Sensory

- Sublenticular part - Auditory radiation to medial geniculate body ⎤ Hearing

  Optic fibres to lateral geniculate body ⎤ Vision

Fig. 3.14
Axial section through L basal ganglia.

Slice 6

This slice (Fig. 3.15) passes through the posterior superior limits of the third ventricle and its immediate posterior relation, the habenular commissure. The roof of the third ventricle is the choroid plexus attached on either side to the stria medullaris thalami. The region immediately above the choroid roof of V3 and bounded laterally by the fornices is known as the velum interpositum. This is usually quite small and traversed by numerous filaments of the pia-arachnoid. Occasionally this region may be an expansive anterior extension of the quadrigeminal plate cistern and is then termed the cavum velum interpositum.

Immediately posterior to the habenular commissure the great vein of Galen is visible (Fig. 3.16). This vein receives paired tributaries of the internal cerebral veins which follow the course of the choroid plexus of the roof of V3 and the paired basal veins of Rosenthal. The great vein of Galen joins with the inferior sagittal sinus to form the straight sinus.

There is calcification in the glomus of the choroid plexus on both sides. The glomus is located in the trigone of each lateral ventricle at the junction of the body with the posterior and temporal horns. Although this calcification is usually symmetrical, unilateral calcification is a recognized normal variation. CT allows detection of calcification in the choroid plexus in 0.5% of patients in the first 10 years of life and the incidence increases steadily after that.

The ventricular system (Fig. 3.17) consists of the paired lateral ventricles (LV) which drain via the foramina of Monro into V3 and then via the cerebral aqueduct of Sylvius into V4. The fourth ventricle drains into the basal cisterns via the midline foramen of Magendie and the lateral foramina of Luschka. CSF subsequently flows through the basal cisterns and over the cerebral convexities to be reabsorbed through the arachnoid granulations of the superior sagittal sinus. Obstruction to the flow of CSF through the ventricles commonly occurs at three sites: foramina of Monro, aqueduct of Sylvius and foramina of Magendie and Luschka.

Anteriorly, the frontal horns of the lateral ventricles are separated by the septum pellucidum.

Posterior to the Sylvian fissure is the superior temporal gyrus containing the sensory area of language (Wernicke's area). More deeply within the cerebral hemisphere and forming the floor of the Sylvian fissure is the transverse temporal gyrus of Heschl which contains the primary auditory cortex.

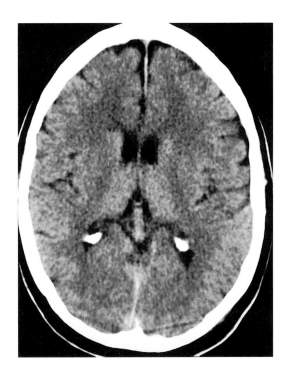

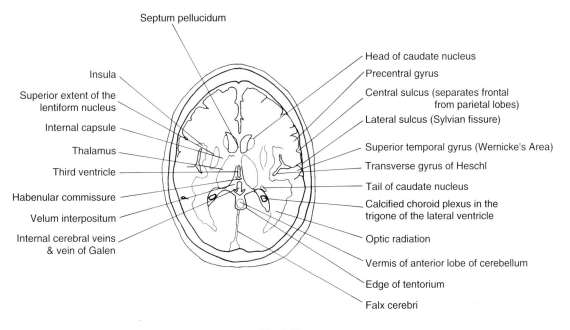

Septum pellucidum

Insula

Superior extent of the
lentiform nucleus

Internal capsule

Thalamus

Third ventricle

Habenular commissure

Velum interpositum

Internal cerebral veins
& vein of Galen

Head of caudate nucleus

Precentral gyrus

Central sulcus (separates frontal
from parietal lobes)

Lateral sulcus (Sylvian fissure)

Superior temporal gyrus (Wernicke's Area)

Transverse gyrus of Heschl

Tail of caudate nucleus

Calcified choroid plexus in the
trigone of the lateral ventricle

Optic radiation

Vermis of anterior lobe of cerebellum

Edge of tentorium

Falx cerebri

Fig. 3.15
Slice 6.

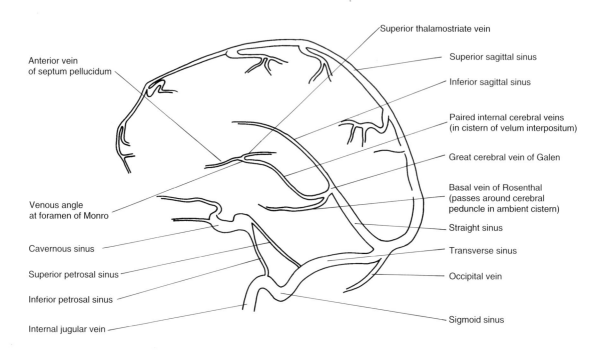

Superior thalamostriate vein

Anterior vein
of septum pellucidum

Superior sagittal sinus

Inferior sagittal sinus

Paired internal cerebral veins
(in cistern of velum interpositum)

Great cerebral vein of Galen

Basal vein of Rosenthal
(passes around cerebral
peduncle in ambient cistern)

Venous angle
at foramen of Monro

Straight sinus

Cavernous sinus

Transverse sinus

Superior petrosal sinus

Occipital vein

Inferior petrosal sinus

Internal jugular vein

Sigmoid sinus

Fig. 3.16
Deep venous drainage of cranium (lateral view).

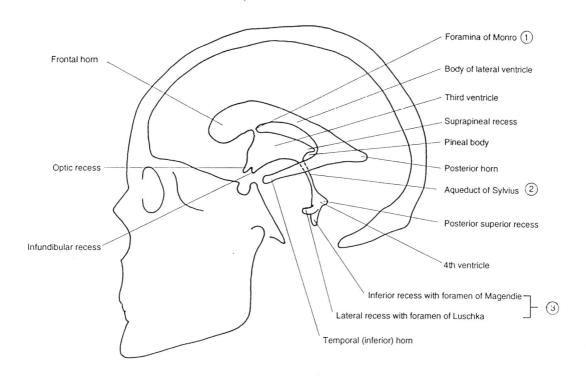

Frontal horn

Optic recess

Infundibular recess

Foramina of Monro ①

Body of lateral ventricle

Third ventricle

Suprapineal recess

Pineal body

Posterior horn

Aqueduct of Sylvius ②

Posterior superior recess

4th ventricle

Inferior recess with foramen of Magendie
Lateral recess with foramen of Luschka ③

Temporal (inferior) horn

Fig. 3.17
Ventricular system.

Slice 7

This slice (Fig. 3.18) passes through the bodies of the lateral ventricles. The fornices form the roof of V3. Posteriorly between the lateral ventricles is the splenium of the corpus callosum which is the major white matter tract connecting the two hemispheres and is divided into three major parts: the genu anteriorly, the body centrally and the splenium posteriorly (Fig. 3.19).

Anteriorly and posteriorly the two cerebral hemispheres are separated by the falx cerebri. The inferior sagittal sinus is seen at the free margin of the posterior falx while the superior sagittal sinus is seen along the calvarial margin of the posterior falx.

Posteriorly on either side of the falx cerebri is the occipital lobe containing the visual cortex. A unilateral lesion here will cause an homonymous hemianopia with a contralateral visual field defect. This should be compared with a lesion involving the optic chiasm which results in a bitemporal hemianopia, whilst a lesion involving the optic nerve anterior to the chiasm results in a scotoma or single eye blindness.

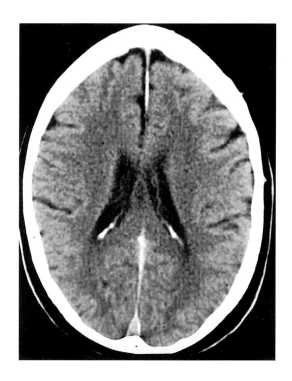

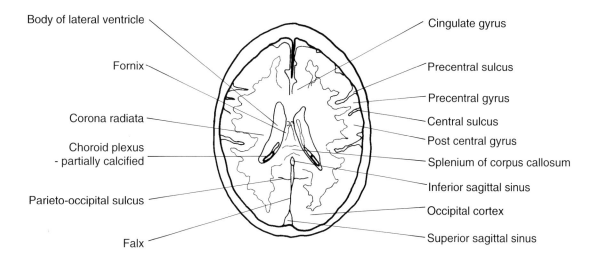

Body of lateral ventricle

Fornix

Corona radiata

Choroid plexus
- partially calcified

Parieto-occipital sulcus

Falx

Cingulate gyrus

Precentral sulcus

Precentral gyrus

Central sulcus

Post central gyrus

Splenium of corpus callosum

Inferior sagittal sinus

Occipital cortex

Superior sagittal sinus

Fig. 3.18
Slice 7.

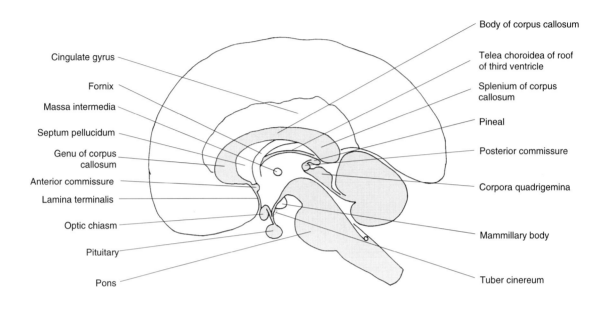

Fig. 3.19
Midline sagittal anatomy.

Slice 8

This slice (Fig. 3.20) and higher slices pass progressively through the superior portions of the cerebral hemispheres. The frontal lobe is separated posteriorly by the central sulcus from the parietal lobe. The primary motor projection cortex is located on the anterior wall of the central (Rolandic) sulcus and the adjacent portion of the precentral gyrus. Cells in this cortex control voluntary movements of skeletal muscle on the opposite side of the body, the impulses travelling along axons in the corticobulbar and corticospinal tracts to the nuclei of the cerebrospinal nerves. There is an inverted relationship within the motor cortex with the lower limb cortex closer to the vertex and the upper limb, hand and face represented progressively more inferiorly toward the Sylvian fissure.

The primary sensory projection cortex for the reception of general sensations is located in the post-central gyrus. It receives fibres from the thalamic radiations conveying skin, muscle, joint and tendon sense from the opposite side of the body. Once again there is topographic organization of the sensory areas in an inverted fashion similar to that seen for the motor cortex. There is, however, considerable overlap in the primary sensory and motor cortex with experimental evidence that a relatively wide portion of the adjacent frontal lobe receives sensory stimuli, whilst motor responses can be achieved by stimulation of the primary sensory areas.

The centrum semi-ovale is the white matter of the telencephalon above the corpus callosum and contains a range of association and projection fibres including fibres to both the sensory and motor cortex. Because of the concentration of white matter at this level, disturbances of grey–white differentiation and selective white matter diseases are often well-appreciated here.

Vascular territories of the brain

Posterior fossa

The arterial supply of the brainstem is divided into medial and lateral territories. The medial territory in the medulla is supplied by anterior spinal arteries, and in the pons by pontine arteries arising directly from the basilar artery. The lateral territory of the medulla is supplied by fine branches of the posterior inferior cerebellar artery and that of the pons by small branches of the anterior inferior cerebellar artery and the superior cerebellar artery. The midbrain is supplied by penetrating branches of the pre-communicating segment of the posterior cerebral artery.

The caudal aspect of the cerebellar hemisphere and cerebellar vermis is supplied by terminal branches of the posterior inferior cerebellar artery (PICA). The anterior inferior cerebellar artery (AICA) also contributes supply to the caudal cerebellar hemisphere as well as supplying the flocculus and the labyrinthine artery to the inner ear. The cranial aspect of the cerebellum is supplied by the superior cerebellar artery.

There is considerable variation in the territories of arterial supply in the posterior fossa, with a reciprocal relationship existing between the AICA and PICA.

Cerebral hemispheres (Fig. 3.21)

In the forebrain there is again a paramedian

Normal anatomy

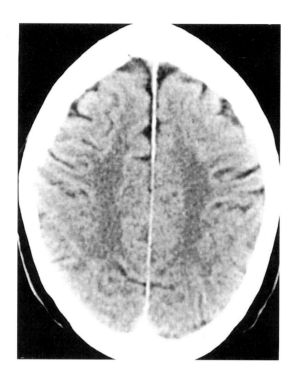

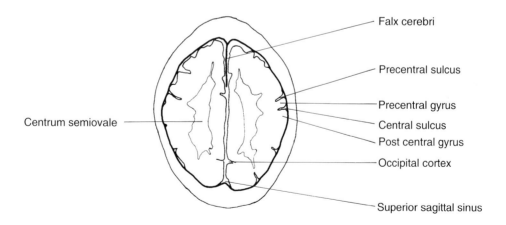

Falx cerebri

Precentral sulcus

Precentral gyrus

Central sulcus

Post central gyrus

Occipital cortex

Superior sagittal sinus

Centrum semiovale

Fig. 3.20
Slice 8.

or central and a lateral or peripheral pattern of distribution of arterial supply, but the vascular territories are far more consistently demarcated. The paramedian region is supplied by small penetrating end arteries arising from the anterior, middle and posterior cerebral arteries. The penetrating branches of the anterior cerebral artery include the recurrent artery of Heubner and medial lenticulostriate arteries, and supply the antero-inferior part of the internal capsule. The penetrating branches of the middle cerebral artery supply most of the putamen and lateral portion of the globus pallidus, superior half of the internal capsule and adjacent corona radiata, and the superior portion of the head and most of the body of the caudate nucleus. The penetrating branches of the posterior cerebral artery supply most of the thalamus, hypothalamus and subthalamic nucleus. Another important penetrating vessel is the anterior choroidal artery which usually arises directly from the internal carotid artery and supplies the posterior two-thirds of the internal capsule, the uncus and amygdaloid nucleus and part of the optic and acoustic radiation.

The peripheral or lateral territories of the cerebral hemispheres are supplied by hemispheric branches of the anterior, middle and posterior cerebral arteries. The anterior cerebral artery (ACA) supplies pericallosal branches to the whole corpus callosum except the splenium, and hemispheric branches to the anterior 75% of the medial surface of the cerebral hemisphere. This includes a 2–3 cm wide strip over the superior cerebral convexity. This supply extends posteriorly as far as the parieto-occipital sulcus medially. On CT slices near the vertex, most of the medial aspect of the cerebral hemispheres is supplied by this vessel, including the primary motor and sensory area of the contralateral leg.

The middle cerebral hemispheric branches supply the insula and the surrounding opercula of the frontal, parietal and temporal lobes to include a large oval territory centred on the Sylvian fissure. On axial CT slices this corresponds roughly to a triangular area demarcated anteriorly and posteriorly by the projection of the frontal and occipital horns of the lateral ventricle to the cortex respectively, a useful and recognizable pattern.

The posterior cerebral artery (PCA), as well as supplying penetrating branches to the thalamus and hypothalamus, supplies hemispheric branches to the inferior and medial aspect of the temporal lobe including the hippocampus, large parts of the medial occipital lobe including the visual cortex and the splenium of the corpus callosum. The anterior extent of supply of the posterior cerebral artery to the temporal lobe should be particularly noted on the accompanying diagram.

The areas of brain lying between two vascular territories are referred to as watershed areas. They are especially vulnerable during episodes of global hypoperfusion. Infarcts in these areas are commonly seen straddling the middle and posterior cerebral arterial territories in the parieto-occipital region. In fact the territory of the anterior cerebral artery is also in contiguity with this area externally. It is thus the only point on the brain surface where the three main vascular territories come into contact. Another vulnerable area exists between the territories supplied by the deep penetrating branches of the middle cerebral artery and its hemispheric branches in a crescentic distribution and in a subinsular location.

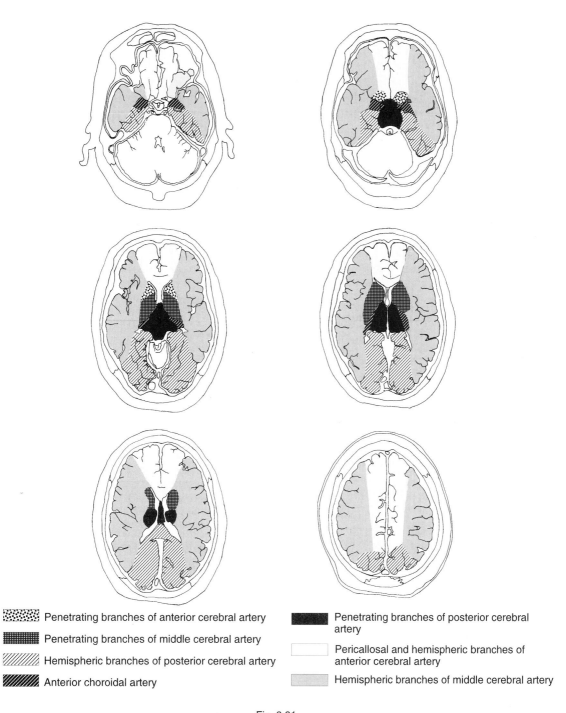

Penetrating branches of anterior cerebral artery

Penetrating branches of middle cerebral artery

Hemispheric branches of posterior cerebral artery

Anterior choroidal artery

Penetrating branches of posterior cerebral artery

Pericallosal and hemispheric branches of anterior cerebral artery

Hemispheric branches of middle cerebral artery

Fig. 3.21
Axial sections from inferior to superior showing the approximate areas of individual vessel supply to the cerebrum.

Bibliography

Chusid J G, McDonald J J 1962 Correlative
neuroanatomy and functional neurology, 11th edn.
Lange, Los Altos

Cormier P J, Long E R, Russell E J 1992 MR Imaging of
posterior fossa infarctions: vascular territories and
clinical correlates. Radiographics 12: 1079–1096

Kretschmann H J, Weinrich W 1986 Neuroanatomy and
cranial computed tomography. Thieme, Stuttgart

Mark L P, Daniels D L, Naidich T P, Brone J A 1993
Limbic system anatomy: an overview. American Journal
of Neuroradiology 14: 349–352

Modic M, Weinstein M A, Rothner A D, Grenberg G,
Duchesneau P M, Kaufman B 1980 Calcification of the
choroid plexus visualized by computed tomography.
Radiology 135: 369–372

Nieuwenhuys R, Voogd J, van Huijzen C 1988 The
human central nervous system, 3rd edn. Springer,
Berlin

Scatliff J H, Clark J K 1992 How the brain got its names
and numbers. American Journal of Neuroradiology 13:
241–248

Schnitzlein H N, Reed Murtagh F 1985 Imaging anatomy
of the head and spine, 2nd edn. Urban and
Schwarzenberg, Munich

CHAPTER 4

The normal scan

i. Approaching the image

General presentation

The initial assessment of any CT scan includes a quick overview of the scanning protocol used, including the use of intravenous contrast medium, and also the detail in which the information has been photographed or displayed. These factors define the limitations of the examination.

The digital nature of the information of the scan may be exploited by performing focal magnification of key areas and by using a variety of window settings as outlined in Chapter 2.

Basic patient identification, unit number and date are usually shown on the top left hand corner of the film. The next image, often photographed adjacent to it, is the scout image or scanning radiograph.

The scout image

The scout image's importance is often underestimated. For those with knowledge of plain film radiology, this is an entirely comparable image with which they can readily identify. Its digital nature allows all the photographic or display variations of a CT slice.

Careful perusal of the scout image is often rewarding. Observation of structural, developmental or bony changes will focus attention to a particular area (Fig. 2.10a; Fig. 4.1).

The scout image may show pathology which would not necessarily have been covered by a standard slice protocol. It may reveal a nasopharyngeal mass, a high cervical spinal abnormality (Fig. 4.2), unsuspected facial pathology, foreign bodies or abnormal collections of air or calcium.

The slices are then prescribed from the scout image. Both the original scout and the annotated version with the slices marked are commonly photographed, as pathology may be less obvious in a heavily annotated image.

The scout film is the key that will link the individual slices into a 3-dimensional unity. It is an invaluable bridge for the observer who is relatively unused to cross-sectional

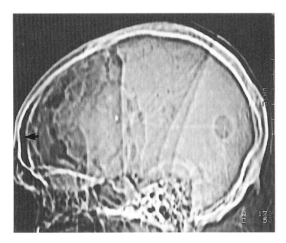

Fig. 4.1
Lateral scout film showing burrhole, craniotomy defect, pneumocephalus (arrow) and ventricular shunt tip.

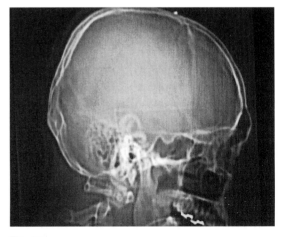

Fig. 4.2
Lateral scout film in patient with recent trauma. No skull fractures are seen, but there is a displaced fracture of the odontoid process.

imaging. Constant marriage of the scout and the individual slices will accelerate the learning process and aid the appreciation of the 3-dimensional structure.

If a patient moves between the scout and the performance of the slice, the value of the scout for localization is reduced. Delay should be minimized at this point of the study.

The slices

CT slices of a head are conventionally displayed in anatomical order, from skull base to vertex, and oriented as though the observer were standing at the foot of the bed.

Each axial image has a relatively small third dimension (slice thickness) and allows a virtual 2-D in 2-D representation. This is unlike conventional radiographs which are essentially a 3-D in 2-D representation in which it is difficult to appreciate contour, separate superimposed structures and appreciate depth of field without a right angled companion image.

Anatomical order and chronological order are not necessarily identical. Sometimes, on the basis of something seen during scanning, additional finer slices may be performed. For photographic purposes, however, they should be recorded in anatomical order so that the eye can flow cleanly through the series in a logical fashion.

Assessment technique

For people accustomed to plain films, the plethora of images presented on CT is at first intimidating. It is a common mistake to begin leaping to conclusions after viewing one or two isolated images, analogous to pronouncing on the contents of the entire Christmas pudding after sampling one or two slices. A serious error which may arise as a consequence of this is the misjudging of the epicentre of a lesion, which causes inaccurate assessment of its origin and extent.

One needs time to scan the images. With practice, this can be rapid, but initially it is useful to look at each CT twice.

On the first quick pass, one simply looks at all the slices in order, to make major observations. Gross pathology is easily observed, and one obtains an overview.

The second pass is more thoughtful, and involves detailed analysis of the abnormalities noted on the first quick glance and the search for other more subtle lesions and ancillary findings. This is where all the fun and challenge of CT interpretation is to be found. It is all about making sense of what has been seen.

ii. Search patterns and initial assessment

Skull

Size

In adult practice, head size is rarely a major consideration. Examination of the scout image should confirm normal cranio-facial proportions and exclude extreme pathology such as microcephaly or acromegaly.

In paediatric practice, with growing calvaria subject to the influences of raised intracranial pressure or premature suture fusion, the assessment is obviously more critical.

Shape and contour

Serial axial scans will reveal most skulls to be oval to round, often with some minor asymmetry at the skull base or the vertex. The scout film will show fractures and other bony abnormalities, but the smaller the lesion the less likely it is to be appreciated on the axial image without wide windowing techniques.

Cross-sectional imaging lends itself to the demonstration of contour deformities of the calvaria, such as depressed fractures (Fig. 4.3), and obviates the need for tangential plain films.

Mineralization

The bones of the skull should be inspected for normal mineralization, as well as a normal diploïc width, and focal areas of bone destruction or sclerosis should be excluded.

Symmetry

Basal and vertical calvarial asymmetry, and the normal variant of plagiocephaly, will produce variations in the symmetry of the intracranial contents. These minor variations are common but should be associated with a normal underlying brain.

Intracranial contents

Symmetry

The intracranial contents generally show a marked tendency to symmetry, with midline structures such as the falx dividing the brain into very similar left and right halves. Any significant deviation from this pattern must be assessed further in terms of the principles outlined in Chapter 5.

Ventriculosulcal proportionality

There is an aesthetically appreciable ventriculo-sulcal proportionality which is more or less preserved through life. In children the ventricles and sulci are small; in adult life both the ventricles and sulci enlarge, but the proportionality should be maintained.

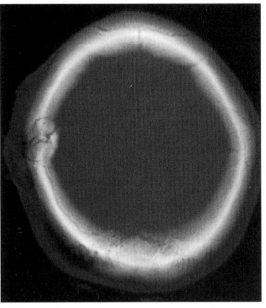

Fig. 4.3 (W2942 C892)
Skull trauma. A wide window photographic technique confirms multiple skull fractures, with depression of an inner table fragment on the right. These details were averaged out on conventional cranial settings. Soft tissue swelling overlies the point of maximal impact.

Within the ventricular system, the lateral, third and fourth ventricles should also be proportional to one another, with any focal increase or decrease in size requiring explanation.

Grey–white differentiation

This also changes with age. In the less myelinated paediatric brain with its higher water content the distinction is more difficult to appreciate. The smaller CSF spaces in children add to the relatively featureless appearance of the paediatric brain.

In the adult, grey–white differentiation is easier to appreciate, but a normal range of appearances must be recognized so that both focal and diffuse abnormalities can be identified. Adult grey matter reads around 40 Hu, which is higher than the 30 Hu of white matter. This is largely because of the fatty myelin in the white matter reducing the average density. Any pathological process which causes the accumulation of lower density material than the normal brain tissue will drop the Hounsfield numbers of the affected area. The accumulation of oedema fluid is a characteristic example. When the tissue affected is predominantly white matter, a common situation in many forms of intracranial pathology producing so-called vasogenic oedema, the effect will be an exaggeration of grey–white differentiation. If however grey matter is predominantly affected, the drop in its Hu will cause a decrease in the normal grey–white contrast, making the brain appear featureless. In rare cases of very severe ischaemia, especially in children, the pattern may even appear to reverse. It is essential to familiarize oneself with the normal grey–white differentiation shown by a particular scanner photographed at standard settings, so that disturbances may be recognized.

The normal scan

Check list

1. Skull
Size, shape, symmetry, mineralization
Focal sclerotic or lytic lesions

2. Ventricles, cisterns and sulci
Ventricles
  Absolute size
  Relative size
Sulci
  Absolute size
  Relative size
Ventriculosulcal proportionality

Identify normal cisterns and fissures esp.
  quadrigeminal plate cistern
  Sylvian fissures

3. Symmetry of intracranial contents
Normal grey–white differentiation
  Identify internal capsules
Exclude midline and bilateral lesions

4. Exclude focal abnormalities
Changes in volume or attenuation; abnormal enhancement

5. Extended search pattern
Orbits, sinuses, nasopharynx, ears, craniocervical junction, face, vault and coverings

6. Technical review
Review appropriateness of slices, projections and photography for the clinical indication

Structuring the report
1. Briefly describe protocol used. This defines the limitations of the study.
2. Make major observations about normal and abnormal structures.
3. Ensure that the clinical issues have been addressed.
4. Correlate with previous imaging to assess natural history of process.
5. List incidental findings and normal variants and put them in clinical perspective.
6. Make recommendations for further imaging or follow up as appropriate.
7. Conclude with a brief summary or impression

CHAPTER 5

The abnormal scan

i. The abnormal skull

Common causes of calvarial thickening, localized hyperostosis and lytic lesions are summarized in Tables 5.1–3. As these are skeletal abnormalites, they often reflect systemic disease, and one should assess the scout image for other manifestations in the cervical spine as well as the facial skeleton, including its modelling and proportionality to the calvarium. In thalassaemia, for example, the thickened calvarium may be accompanied by hypoplastic paranasal sinuses as these too are recruited for extramedullary blood element production.

Table 5.1
Common causes of calvarial thickening

Congenital/developmental
  Fibrous dysplasia, other less common
    skeletal syndromes
Neoplastic
  Osteoblastic metastases
  Myelosclerosis
Metabolic/systemic
  Extramedullary haemopoeisis
  Acromegaly
  Abnormal calcium and phosphorus metabolism
Miscellaneous
  Paget's disease
Iatrogenic
  Phenytoin ingestion
  Fluorosis

Table 5.2
Localized calvarial density or hyperostosis

Developmental
  – Hemiatrophy with local bony overgrowth
  – Fibrous dysplasia
Neoplastic
  – Sclerotic metastases (prostate and breast)
  – Meningioma
  – Primary bone tumours
Miscellaneous
  – Frontal hyperostosis
  – Paget's disease

Table 5.3
**Common lytic skull lesions
(Single or multiple)**

Congenital/developmental
  – Normal variants including parietal foramina,
    focal thinning, etc.
  – Benign lesions including dermoids, epidermoids
  – Meningocele, encephalocele
Neoplastic
  – Metastatic (breast, lung, thyroid, kidney)
  – Multiple myeloma/plasmacytoma
  – Direct extension from intracranial, scalp, sinus
    or nasopharyngeal tumours
Traumatic
  – Burr hole, craniotomy
Inflammatory, infective
  – Cholesteatoma
  – Osteomyelitis
Miscellaneous
  – Fibrous dysplasia
  – Histiocytosis X
  – Paget's disease/osteoporosis circumscripta
  – Metabolic diseases including
    hyperparathyroidism

ii. Disturbances in ventricular size; ventriculo-sulcal proportionality and appropriateness for age

The ventricles are readily appreciated on any CT image because of the contrast between their CSF content and the brain. In perceptual terms, therefore, they often hold the key to analysing the image, whether it is due to primary pathology in the ventricles, or the secondary expression upon the ventricular system of pathology in the adjacent brain.

Global ventricular enlargement
(Table 5.4)

Ventricles which are large for age must generally be viewed with concern. CT has taught care in the use of the term 'hydrocephalus' as opposed to the simple observation of ventricular enlargement. True hydrocephalus implies

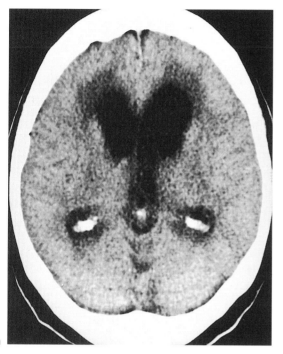 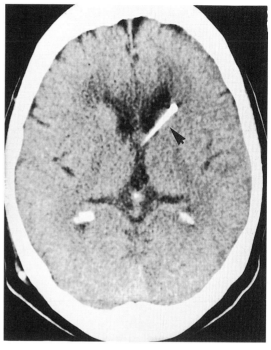

a   b

Fig. 5.1 a & b
(a) Obstructive hydrocephalus. There is loss of ventriculosulcal proportionality with large ventricles and no visible peripheral sulci. A haze of periventricular oedema is noticeable especially around the frontal horns.**(b) Same patient, 11 days later, after insertion of shunt (arrow).** Ventriculosulcal proportionality has been restored, with a reduction in ventricular size, and reappearance of the Sylvian fissures and cortical sulci. The periventricular oedema has reduced.

a disturbance in the complex dynamics of CSF production or flow, or both, and frequently needs neurosurgical intervention. When a state of dysequilibrium exists due to

Table 5.4
Enlarged cerebral ventricles

> **Obstructive/non-communicating hydrocephalus**
>   Pattern depends on site of obstruction
> **Non-obstructive/communicating hydrocephalus**
>   Usually involves subarachnoid space pathology
> **Dilatation ex vacuo**
>   Loss/atrophy of adjacent brain tissue
> **Overproduction of CSF**
>   Choroid stimulation following subarachnoid
>   haemorrhage
>   Choroid plexus papillomas

increased production of CSF, impaired drainage and circulation or acute focal obstruction, pressure rises within the ventricles, and fluid may accumulate in the periventricular interstitium. Observation of this blurred periventricular halo is a sign that equilibrium has not been reached (Fig. 5.1).

'Hydrocephalus' may enlarge ventricles to a point, and then arrest, as compensatory mechanisms come into play and a new equilibrium is reached. Big ventricles may thus no longer be under pressure and may not necessarily need shunting.

Ventricles which are under pressure will show changes in shape, such as rounding of the frontal horns, prominence of the temporal horns or bulging of the walls of the third ventricle. The ventricular margins appear tight and stretched. Given increasing time and severity the raised intraventricular pressure will be communicated through the overlying brain with concomitant sulcal effacement.

When all four ventricles are distended and in free communication the surface pathways are presumed to have been damaged. This is a common paediatric pattern and may follow meningitis. It may also be seen in adults with inflammation or neoplastic infiltration of the meninges, and after subarachnoid haemorrhage. Occasionally obstruction to the exit foramina of V4 can produce dilatation of all four ventricles, mimicking a communicating pattern, but this can be clarified by isotope studies.

The second common mechanism for ventricular enlargement is central atrophy. Gliosis, withering or atrophy of central brain tissue will cause ventricular dilatation ex vacuo, and will often be accompanied by low attenuation change in the periventricular white matter, which will be more sharply marginated and often lower in density than interstitial or periventricular oedema (Fig. 5.2). Distinguishing between periventricular oedema and periventricular gliosis is of paramount importance. Failure to do so may explain the disappointing results of some shunting procedures, where the presence of unrecognized permanent white matter damage has limited the patient's improvement after surgery. If doubt exists, CSF transport studies should be accompanied by direct ventricular pressure monitoring prior to shunt insertion.

Globally enlarged ventricles and prominent sulci may be seen in conditions producing 'reversible atrophy' such as alcoholism,

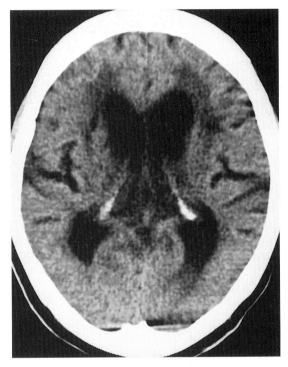

Fig. 5.2
Central atrophy due to white matter ischaemia has allowed dilatation of the ventricles. Intraventricular pressure is not increased.

starvation, anorexia nervosa and the administration of catabolic steroids.

Focal ventricular enlargement

Developmental variations
Focal enlargement of the occipital horns or colpocephaly is seen as part of the constellation of abnormalities seen in conditions such as agenesis of the corpus callosum (Fig. 5.9) and should not be mistaken for acquired pathology requiring treatment.

Congenital abnormalities
Aqueduct stenosis due to congenital forking or gliosis will produce selective dilatation of

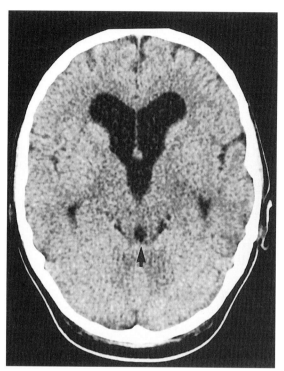

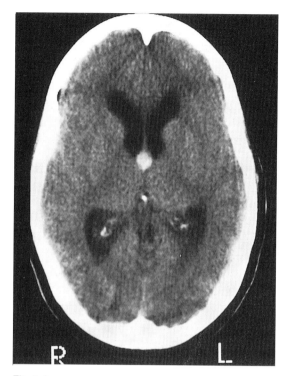

Fig. 5.3
Aqueduct stenosis in asymptomatic 37-year-old woman. The lateral and third ventricles are enlarged, as is the proximal aqueduct (arrow). On the next slice, inferiorly, the stenotic point was reached and the aqueduct was no longer identifiable. The intracranial equilibrium has been re-established, as is shown by the absence of periventricular oedema, and the presence of identifiable Sylvian fissures.

Fig. 5.4
Plain scan showing hyperdense colloid cyst producing selective dilatation of the lateral ventricles

the lateral and third ventricles as shown in Figure 5.3. The thickness of the cortical mantle does not necessarily correlate with anticipated post shunt recovery for the individual case. In aqueduct stenosis the frontal horns may appear to have been relatively spared, but the discrepant dilatation of the occipital horns often remits after shunting.

Acquired

Strategically placed obstructing lesions such as colloid cysts of the third ventricle may cause focal dilatation of the lateral ventricles.

This is a distinctive pattern (Fig. 5.4). Colloid cysts are commonly different in density from surrounding brain but occasionally isodense, making it necessary to recognize the pattern of obstruction.

It is important to scrutinize the third and especially the fourth ventricles, where an obstructing cysticercal cyst or cystic neoplasm may be mistaken for the ventricle itself. The cyst contents usually have an attenuation value higher than CSF (Fig. 5.44).

A ventricle may enlarge focally if it abuts an area of profoundly softened or atrophic brain (Fig. 5.5). This is the ex vacuo mechanism at work again. This may be seen for example as the sequel to severe subependymal haemorrhage in the premature infant but

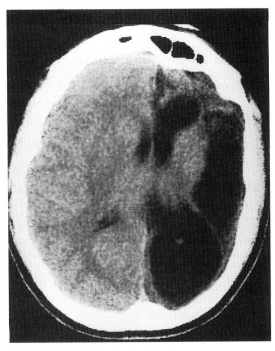 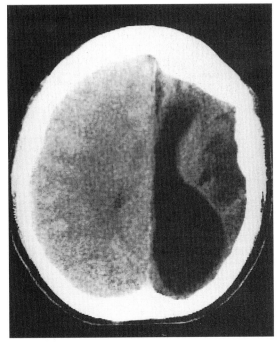

Fig. 5.5
An ischaemic insult in childhood has resulted in failure of normal growth in the left hemisphere. The falx is displaced to the left but not bowed. The left lateral ventricle has ballooned to occupy the space created by the damaged brain, which shows encephalomalacia so profound it approaches CSF density. There is also focal calvarial thickening on the higher slice.

can follow many other insults. Commonly the expanded area of CSF density can be appreciated as part of the ventricle, and is in free communication with it. Sometimes it may become sequestered and form a porencephalic cyst. Manipulating the window may help appreciate the presence or absence of a wall in this case.

Globally small ventricles

This is a normal state of affairs in the paediatric age group, where ventricles are slit-like.

In adulthood a spectrum of appearances exists but the tendency is for ventricles to enlarge with age, with reduction in the brain turgor and the accrual of small ischaemic

insults with subsequent loss of brain tissue. Small ventricles therefore in a patient over, for example, 60 years, should prompt a careful assessment of the cerebral sulci to see whether proportionality has been maintained, and also of the cerebral parenchyma for signs of swelling to suggest active pathology. In younger patients where the ventricles are normally expected to be smaller, assessment of grey–white differentiation becomes even more crucial in deciding whether the small ventricles are associated with pathology (Fig. 5.6). Major causes of diffuse brain swelling which could produce a picture of globally small ventricles are shown in Table 5.5.

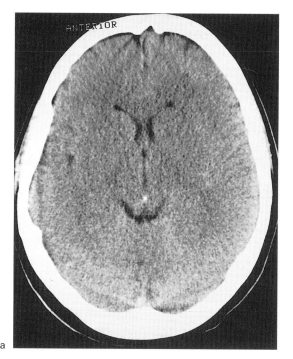

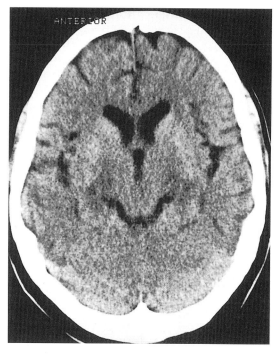

a   b

Fig. 5.6 a & b
(a) This young woman was in diabetic ketoacidotic coma and was unconscious for days before being found. The ventricles are slit-like due to the diffuse brain swelling, and normal grey–white differentiation was lost at this standard photographic setting (W72, C37).
(b) Ten days later the swelling has subsided, restoring grey–white differentiation, but atrophy is already present, with ventricles and sulci inappropriately large for age. The patient was left significantly disabled.

Table 5.5
Diffuse brain swelling

Metabolic/anoxic
  Anoxia
  Hypertension
  Renal or liver failure
  Other profound metabolic disturbances

Infective
  Encephalitis

Miscellaneous
  Head trauma
  Superior sagittal sinus thrombosis
  Pseudotumour cerebri

Focally small ventricles

It is abnormal to see one of the ventricles significantly smaller than the others. If this is observed, a local mass lesion compressing the ventricle should be sought. In the case of a fourth ventricle disproportionately smaller than the others, the cause is usually obstruction to the aqueduct, though the fourth may show relative sparing in other conditions such as normal pressure hydrocephalus. Although the aqueduct is small, its course should be carefully traced down the brain stem, and deviations in course or changes in calibre excluded.

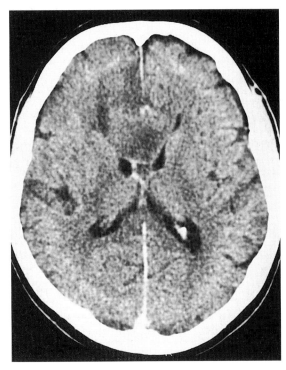

Fig. 5.7
Midline frontal glioma causing symmetrical compression of the frontal horns against the caudate nuclei. The low density of the tumour, and the splaying and posterior displacement of the ventricles distinguish this from ependymal coarctation.

Table 5.6
Enhancing ventricular margins

Inflammatory
 Ventriculitis

Systemic malignancy
 Disseminated non-Hodgkin's lymphoma,
  leukaemia
 Meningeal carcinomatosis (small cell carcinoma
  of lung, melanoma, breast carcinoma)

Subependymal spread of primary CNS neoplasm
 Ependymal spread or seeding from glioma,
  medulloblastoma, germinoma
 Primary CNS lymphoma

Occasionally the frontal horns may show focal coarctation as a result of adherent ependyma. This is usually not of clinical significance, but should be differentiated from focal compression by a tumour (Fig. 5.7).

Ventricular encasement and periventricular enhancement

The ventricular margins should also be assessed (Table 5.6). Inflammatory processes within the ventricle can thicken the ventricular wall which will enhance with intravenous contrast. Occasionally the ventricular wall will appear stiff and even lumpy, an appearance which is nearly always hyperdense to surrounding brain on plain scans, and which enhances dramatically. This may be due to a primary 'butterfly' glioma spreading through the corpus callosum to encase the ventricles, or to transependymal spread of other CNS neoplasms (Fig. 5.8).

General ventricular disorganization

The most severe developmental disorders producing bizarre ventricular dispositions, such as holoprosencephaly, are usually diagnosed in the paediatric age group. Less severe conditions, especially if isolated, may present unexpectedly in later life. The most common of these to cause a recognizable disorganization of normal ventricular relationships is agenesis of the corpus callosum (AGCC), where the patient's disability may be limited to a disconnection effect leading to a tactile aphasia. CT shows disproportionately small frontal horns, separated by the abnormally high-riding third ventricle (Fig. 5.9). The ventricular bodies run an unusually parallel course, separated by

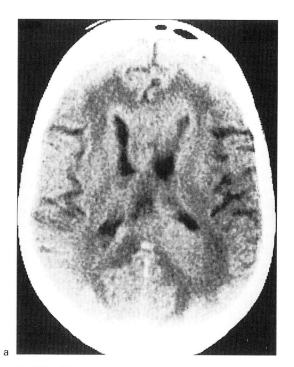
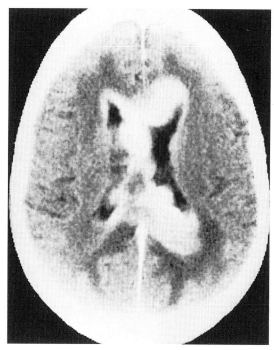

a

b

Fig. 5.8 a & b
Plain (a) and enhanced (b) scans of patient with ventricular encasement by metastatic medulloblastoma.

Probst bundles instead of being linked superiorly by the normal commissural fibres. Colpocephaly or occipital horn dilatation is part of the syndrome.

Sagittal reformations can clarify developmental abnormalities of the fourth ventricle and related midline structures, as in the Dandy–Walker malformation where hypoplasia and malrotation of the vermis is associated with a 'roofless' fourth ventricle opening dorsally into a cyst. The recognition of a normal vermis will also help distinguish arachnoid cysts and large cisternae magnae from this condition and its variants.

With time and practice, however, one becomes able to perform a mental integration of slices taken in one plane only, in such a way as to provide ready understanding of the shape and location of any pathology. All slice based imaging interpretation should be approached with the development of this skill in mind. Training the eye to flow through all the slices containing the abnormality is the key step in the process. The ground the slices cover is governed by their number and thickness, and one needs a sense of this to gauge the third dimension. Abnormalities which involve displacement in the vertical plane, such as the third ventricle in AGCC, test this perception skill to the limit. Subtle antero-posterior displacements, such as the posterior displacement of the fourth ventricle or aqueduct by an infiltrated or swollen brainstem, are difficult for the same reason, in that the displaced structure has a vertical orientation. Assessments such as these must be done consciously until they become second nature.

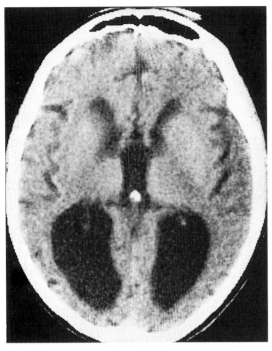 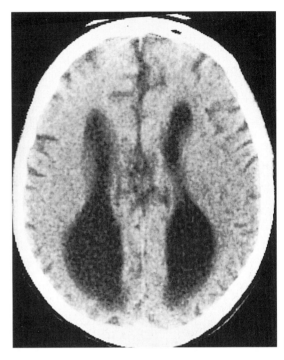

a

b

Fig. 5.9 a & b
Agenesis of corpus callosum.

Ventricular shunting

Surgical shunting may produce rapid ventricular collapse with subdural haematoma formation or be complicated by infection, periventricular cyst formation or CSF loculation (Fig. 5.10). In successful cases, the periventricular oedema may take time to subside, especially if remyelination of damaged fibres is required.

Asymmetric ventricles

Apart from the pathologic conditions discussed above, there also exists a common normal variation which produces asymmetry between the paired left and right lateral ventricles.

It may be that the patient is in an asynclitic or skewed position and that the axial slice does not pass through the same level on the two sides. Even if the patient is well positioned, marked plagiocephaly will disturb symmetry. However, even in the normally shaped and positioned head, minor degrees of asymmetry may still be observed between the lateral ventricles (Fig. 5.11). This is extremely common and generally of no clinical consequence, but the adjacent brain should be carefully inspected for any focal atrophy or infiltrative process which could alter the dynamics of the ventricular walls before affecting the midline structures. In particular, the contrast offered by the normal grey and white matter with structures such as the internal capsule and the corona radiata

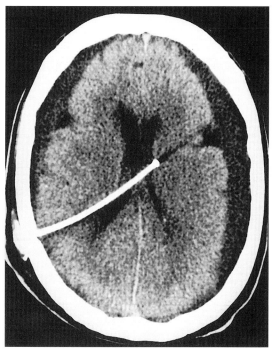

Fig. 5.10
**Rapid decompression of hydrocephalus by a
ventricular shunt has resulted in the development of
symmetrical chronic subdural hygromas.** The cortex is
displaced from the inner table, and the sulci do not gape,
distinguishing this appearance from the enlarged
subarachnoid space seen in atrophy.

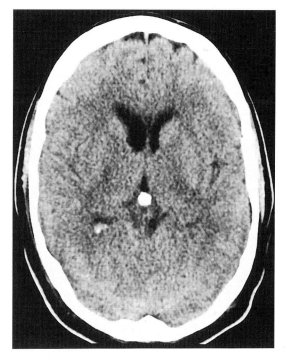

Fig. 5.11
Ventricular asymmetry as a normal variant. The
presence of symmetric internal capsule structures
indicates normal adjacent brain.

should be assessed. If these are normal, it is
unlikely that a mass lesion is present to
account for the ventricular asymmetry.
Besides, the asymmetry is usually across a
broad front. This means that a mass lesion
with this circumference or border would
have to be large in size, and should be easily
detectable on other grounds.

Ventriculosulcal proportionality

Ventricles and sulci should always be
assessed together because they are linked in
the expression of pathology.

Large ventricles and small sulci suggest

hydrocephalus or central atrophy; smaller
ventricles with large sulci suggest ventricular
compression or, more commonly, peripheral
atrophy. Atrophy may be associated with
presenile dementia but the clinical correlation is unreliable in individual cases.

Sulcal size should also be of a harmonious
pattern within the skull. Where selective
atrophy has occurred within a compartment
it is commonly in the posterior fossa with
syndromes such as olivopontocerebellar degeneration, or with alcohol abuse, paraneo-
plastic syndromes and the phenytoin/seizure
combination. In these conditions V4 is commonly enlarged too, but the supratentorial
compartment is relatively spared.

Occasionally the ventricles appear normal

for age, with the abnormality confined to the sulci. Excluding the developmental abnormalities such as lissencephaly, pachygyria and polymicrogyria, focal sulcal abnormalities usually reflect adjacent pathology. Acute swelling effaces sulci, and atrophy causes them to gape. Swelling of meninges or other surface pathology may obscure the sulci.

The sulci over the vertex should always be inspected for asymmetry which may be an early expression of hemisphere swelling.

iii. The focal intracranial lesion

The evaluation of focal intracranial pathology constitutes the major challenge in the assessment of CT head scans in an average patient population. Focal lesions are usually more obvious than diffuse lesions, because of the disturbance of symmetry they cause. All should clearly be approached with knowledge of the clinical context, including age and gender of the patient, and nature and duration of symptoms.

If focal lesions are analysed in terms of the following approach, a broad diagnostic category can be reached which will be sufficient for immediate management decisions.

Location

Precise location is arguably the single most important parameter of any focal intracranial lesion, where the old adage of 'if you know where it is, you know what it is' holds true. It holds good for tumours and for many other categories of pathology.

The first vital distinction is between intra- and extra-axial pathology.

Extra-axial pathology

Extra-axial pathology arises in structures adjacent to the brain surface, such as cranial nerves or meninges, and is usually relatively benign histologically and behaviourally. Tumours tend to be well-differentiated, with a few exceptions, and the effects of the focal lesion are related mainly to local mass and compression of cortex and cranial nerves. Neurosurgery for extra-axial masses has a higher success rate and fewer complications. All efforts should be made to classify a lesion as extra-axial or intra-axial, including MR and carotid angiography where necessary. Lesions which produce dural reaction or invasion, and obtain a blood supply from the external carotid artery are likely to be extra-axial, though exceptions exist.

Anatomically, extra-axial lesions may be considered as convexity or basal in location. Convexity lesions include extracerebral collections and arachnoid cysts, the latter favouring the anterior and middle cranial fossae, though they may be seen in all areas of arachnoid reflection, including the tentorial hiatus. There may be clues to congenital origin, in the form of hypoplasia of the adjacent temporal lobe, or local bony changes. Generally speaking, changes to adjacent bone are far more likely to occur with extra-axial lesions, though, rarely, indolent intra-axial neoplasms may scallop the overlying calvarium.

Of the extra-axial tumours, meningiomas are the most common, and are frequently multiple. Sites of predilection include all dural reflections such as the falx and tentorium, and also the sphenoid ridge (where bone changes are especially common), planum sphenoidale and cerebellopontine angle. The tumour is often sessile, producing a characteristic D-shaped mass. Useful clues to the extra-axial location include the identification of a thin film of CSF between the mass and

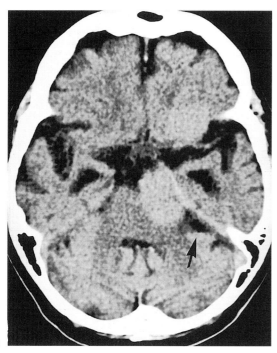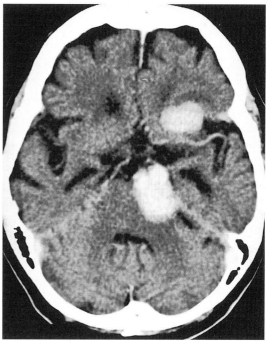

a

b

Fig. 5.12 a & b
(a) Precontrast and (b) postcontrast study of patient with 2 meningiomas, demonstrating the widening of the L cerebellopontine angle as a clue to the extra-axial location (arrow). The tumours are sharply circumscribed, homogeneously hyperdense to brain, and diffusely, strongly enhancing. Note the deformity of the grey–white junction in the L frontal lobe as a clue to the presence of the smaller lesion.

the brain surface, and buckling away of the adjacent brain with displacement of the grey–white junction and widening of adjacent cisterns (Fig. 5.12).

A useful hint to the origin of any focal lesion is to find its epicentre. Many tumours follow a concentric growth pattern. An intelligent guess can be made as to a tumour epicentre by perusal of the slice where it reaches its greatest diameter. This also prevents the error of looking at a slice through the periphery of a mass, where it invaginates into brain and appears to be surrounded by parenchyma on all surfaces, and erroneously ascribing it an intra-axial origin (Fig. 5.13). Special care should be taken with vascular abnor-

malities, such as vertebrobasilar dolichoectasia (VBDE) or giant aneurysms, which may burrow deeply into adjacent tissue and give a false impression of their origins. Recognition of a tubular or fusiform shape should suggest a vascular lesion.

In the CP angle the main diagnosis rests between meningioma and acoustic Schwannoma, though other lesions occur (Table 5.7). Centring on and extension of a tumour into the IAC clearly favours acoustic Schwannoma, as does erosive change to the bony canal. The anatomic relationship to the tentorium is well shown in coronal views, especially where a posterior fossa lesion projects above the level of the petrous ridge in

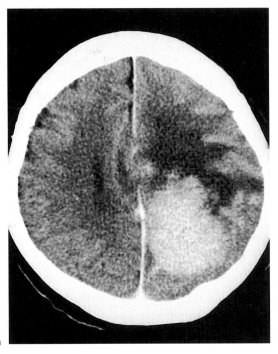

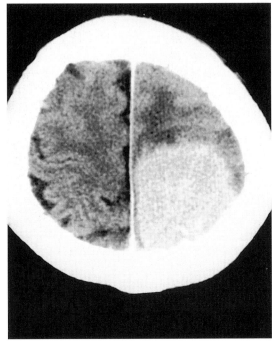

a   b

Fig. 5.13 a & b
(a) and (b) Enhanced scans near the vertex of the same patient, with magnification of the higher slice (b). At the periphery of the lesion, the tumour appears to be surrounded by brain (intra-axial), but the slice through the centre of the lesion (b) shows its epicentre to be much closer to the vertex, and its origin dural. Diagnosis: meningioma.

Table 5.7
Cerebellopontine angle masses

Normal
    Prominent flocculus
Developmental
    Epidermoid
    Arachnoid cyst
Neoplasms
    Acoustic Schwannoma
    Meningioma
Vascular
    Aneurysm, vascular ectasia of vertebral, basilar or
        inferior cerebellar aneurysm

the angled axial image (Fig. 2.8). The presence of hyperostosis favours meningioma, and bone windows should be used to exploit this distinction (Fig. 5.14).

A pineal location of a mass (Fig. 5.75) narrows it essentially to a tumour of germ cell origin or pineal origin, though metastases and lesions of maldevelopment such as dermoids and epidermoids also occur.

There is, morphologically, considerable overlap between pineal lesions in terms of size, composition and enhancement patterns, so demographic data become most important. Germinomas account for over half of primary pineal neoplasms and are usually seen in young adult males. Pineal cell origin tumours are most commonly seen in the form of pineocytomas in young girls.

Basal extra-axial lesions include other neurogenic lesions, some of which are extremely specific in location such as Schwannomas

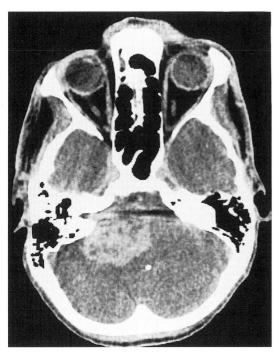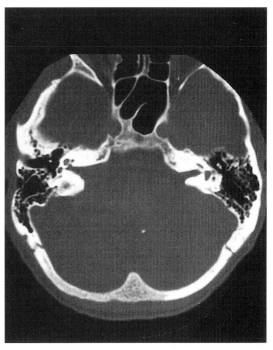

a   b

Fig. 5.14 a & b
(a) Enhanced scan (W300, C54) of CP angle tumour. (b) Bony window (W4000, C668) shows that although the canal appears flared, there is hyperostosis of the posterior lip, an appearance favouring meningioma over acoustic Schwannoma.

involving the trigeminal ganglion (Fig. 5.15). Schwannomas generally favour sensory nerves. Vascular lesions such as giant aneurysms must be included, as well as sellar and parasellar pathology (See Midline lesions).

A special category of extra-axial pathology is the group of conditions showing transcranial spread. Frequently these are tumours which have started in the skull, such as metastatic lesions (Fig. 5.16), or have crossed through the skull as part of their preferred growth vectors. Nasopharyngeal carcinoma has a penchant for perineural spread, and follows the natural foramina in the skull base to gain cranial access, while olfactory neuroblastoma erodes directly through the cribri-form plate to reach the anterior cranial fossa. Lymphoma too is no respecter of boundaries (Fig. 5.17). Wherever transcranial spread is suspected it is again essential to try and identify the epicentre of the process, and to continue scanning in both superior and inferior directions until one is well clear of the process. Because of their frequent cranial nerve presentations, for example, patients with nasopharyngeal carcinoma may have a cranial study as the first diagnostic step, and it is tragic if the inferior extent of the lesion is missed. Bone windows are mandatory in transcranial pathology, and may be informative as to the degree of aggression of the process. An extended field of view in the vertical dimension is provided by coronal

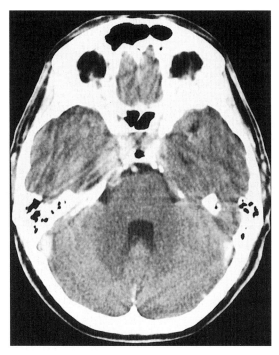

Fig. 5.15
Solid dumb-bell-shaped tumour related to the trigeminal ganglion. The epicentre is Meckel's cave. The posterior extra-axial component has widened the R CP angle. The solid and enhancing nature of this tumour distinguishes it from other bilobed lesions at the petrous tip such as epidermoid cysts, which are of fluid density.

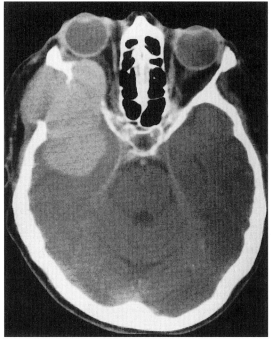

Fig. 5.16
Enhanced scan showing metastatic malignant fibrous histiocytoma. The tumour showed unusually slow and orderly growth, and has smoothly eroded the temporal squama and the greater wing of sphenoid, to cause proptosis, which was the presenting symptom.

images which will also clarify the relationship of the process to the skull base.

Infectious processes such as petrous cholesteatomas and paranasal sinus mucoceles may also have transcranial manifestations as a result of bone destruction and are dealt with further in Chapter 7. Less destructive infectious processes may reach the cranium from the face through the normal rich transcranial vascular connections such as those in the pterygopalatine fossa. Systemic conditions such as histiocytosis X may show both intra- and extra-axial manifestations.

Intra-axial pathology

Once a lesion has been classified as intra-axial, the prognosis is frequently more serious and the surgery more difficult. Lesions arising within the neuraxis are freer to spread than those outside, and are more likely to provoke oedema which aggravates symptoms.

Features which point directly to a lesion being intra-axial include spread across the corpus callosum (Fig. 5.18) or thickening of the septum pellucidum. This must be distinguished from severe focal oedema caused by subfalcine herniation.

The abnormal scan

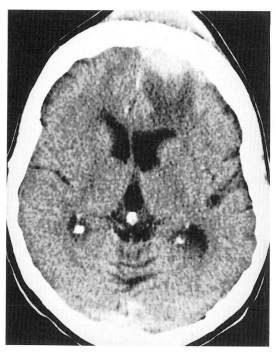

a

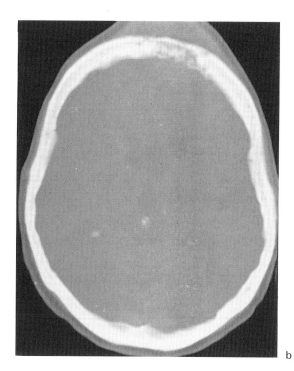

b

Fig. 5.17 a & b
Lymphoma showing transcranial spread. The tumour
has enhanced diffusely. The bony window (b) (W1836,
C71) shows an aggressive, permeative pattern of bone
destruction typical of non-Hodgkin's lymphoma.

Fig. 5.18   (*below right*)
**Enhanced scan showing spread of R occipital glioma
across the splenium of the corpus callosum.**

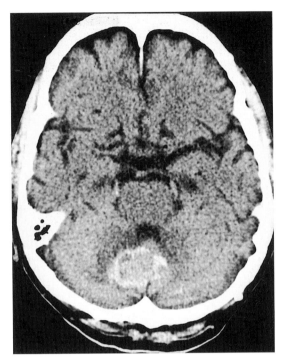

Fig. 5.19
Unenhanced scan showing calcified cerebellar metastasis from mucin-secreting colonic carcinoma.

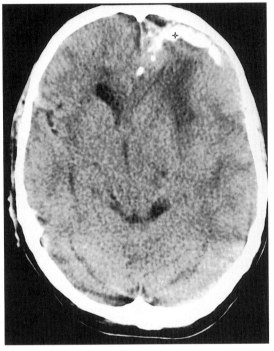

Fig. 5.20
Classic frontal location of oligodendroglioma, with coarse, craggy L frontal calcification.

Even within the neuraxis, some broad anatomic predilections emerge: gliomas and metastases often grow at the grey–white junction where both abrupt vessel calibre changes and biochemical changes occur. Diseases such as multiple sclerosis clearly favour white matter, and are dealt with in more detail later. There are lobar and compartmental preferences as well, with the posterior fossa being a favoured site for childhood astrocytoma, medulloblastoma, ependymoma and haemangioma, though metastases remain the commonest cerebellar tumour in adults (Fig. 5.19).

The frontal lobe is favoured by oligoden-drogliomas (Fig. 5.20) and also by conditions such as Pick's disease, whereas the temporal lobe is the invariable starting point for herpes simplex encephalitis (HSE).

Table 5.8 lists conditions favouring an intraventricular location (Fig. 5.21) and Table 5.9 those with a penchant for involving the corpus callosum.

Shape is usually the most useful identifying feature of an infarct, but location runs it a close second. Knowledge of vascular territories and their watershed areas is often sufficient to enable a confident diagnosis of an ischaemic lesion on location alone (Fig. 5.22), or to exclude one (Fig. 5.23).

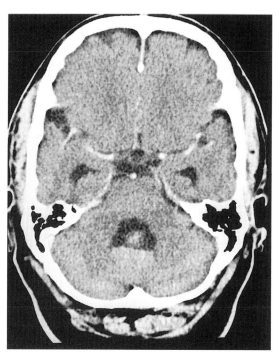

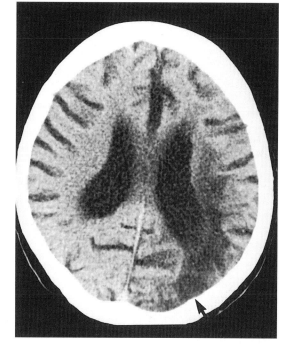

Fig. 5.21   (*above left*)
**Enhanced scan showing small ependymoma within
the fourth ventricle.** The temporal horns are beginning
to dilate as a result of early obstructive hydrocephalus in
this young patient.

Fig. 5.22   (*above right*)
**Classic watershed infarct (arrow) involving a wedge-
shaped region between middle and posterior cerebral
artery territories.** In fact, viewed from the lateral surface
of the brain, this is also a watershed between the anterior
cerebral artery and the MCA and PCA, making this
particular wedge of tissue uniquely vulnerable. Further
infarction of the watershed type extends along the margin
of the L lateral ventricle.

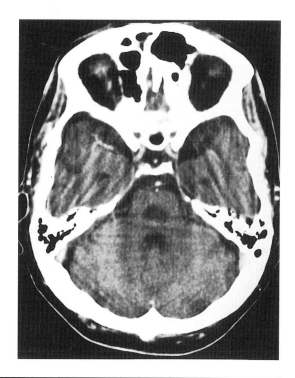

Fig. 5.23   (*right*)
**Central pontine myelinolysis, associated with
hyponatraemia and alcoholism.** The central location of
this characteristic low density triangular lesion is
inconsistent with the patterns of ischaemia in this region
which are usually lateralized.

Table 5.8
Lateral ventricular neoplasms

Under 5 years
  Choroid plexus papilloma
  Primitive neurectodermal tumour (PNET)
  Teratoma
Children and young adults
  Low grade glioma
  Subependymal giant cell astrocytoma (SGCA)
Adults over 30
  Meningioma
  Subependymoma
  Glioblastoma
  Lymphoma
  Metastasis

Table 5.9
Lesions affecting the corpus callosum

Neoplastic
  Gliomas
  Lymphoma
Demyelinating
  Multiple sclerosis
  Acute disseminated encephalomyelitis (ADEM)
  Progressive multifocal leukoencephalopathy (PML)
  Marchiafava–Bignami syndrome

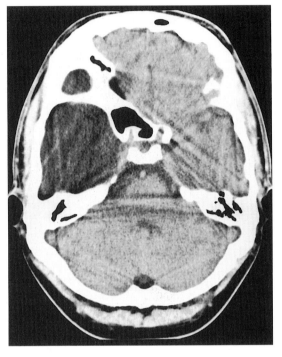

Fig. 5.24
R middle cranial fossa arachnoid cyst with overgrowth and florid pneumatization of the ipsilateral anterior clinoid. Slices at more inferior levels in this patient showed enlargement of the fossa with thinning of the bone.

Making space or taking space

Evaluation of a focal intracranial lesion in terms of whether it is associated with atrophy ('making' or creating space) or space occupation is also of vital importance.

Space-creating lesions

A lesion which 'makes' or creates space implies that there has been irreversible damage to a structure, causing it to shrink. It no longer occupies its normal allocated volume. Since nature abhors a vacuum, the space which has been created is filled by additional CSF if the process is near the surface, or by compensatory dilatation of part of an adjacent ventricle. Such focal ventricular enlargement may be as a result of the CSF

pulsations not encountering the anticipated resistance of adjacent brain with normal turgor.

Other structures may grow to fill up this additional space, especially in the young patient where remodelling is far more easily achieved than in the mature cranium with its fused sutures. The contralateral hemisphere will appear hypertrophied, if the insult has occurred at the time of craniocerebral growth and development. Bone may thicken focally, or nearby paranasal sinuses become overdeveloped. Increased pneumatization of clinoid processes or petrous tips are further examples consistent with a lack of normal

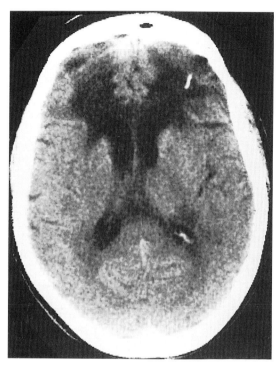

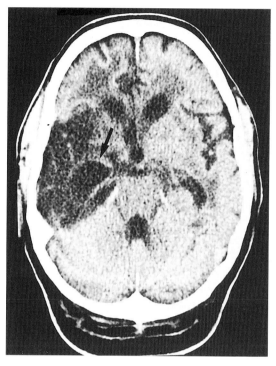

Fig. 5.25
Plain scan in patient with previous pre-frontal leukotomy. There is hypodensity confined to the frontal lobe white matter, and volume loss as shown by the selective ballooning of the frontal horns. A fleck of dystrophic calcification is present on the L.

Fig. 5.26
Atrophy in a characteristic location. The emphasis here is in the R temporal lobe which contains a passively dilated temporal horn (arrow). Minor changes were present in the frontal lobes and in the L temporal lobe on other slices. This profound temporal gliosis should always suggest the sequelae of herpes simplex encephalitis.

brain nearby and consequent loss of the stimuli associated with its perfusion and pulsation (Fig. 5.24).

A lesion associated with focal atrophy is generally old and seldom requires active management. Examples include gliosis (microcystic encephalomalacia) following trauma or surgery, old infarction and any other process which has resulted in irreversible focal damage and scarring. Such old lesions will not enhance with intravenous contrast. In addition, they may show signs of dystrophic calcification and their location may be characteristic of specific pathology (Figs 5.25, 5.26).

Space-occupying lesions

A lesion which occupies space locally, which causes focal swelling, displaces structures away from itself and exhibits mass effect, is a cause for immediate concern.

Sulci, ventricles and cisterns will show pressure effects and effacement. In this context inspection of the sulci over the vertex, on the highest slices, may give the earliest evidence that a space-occupying process is present. Flattening or loss of the normal 'grin' of the quadrigeminal plate cistern (cf Chapter 2) may be the earliest sign of swelling in the brain stem or cerebellum. The Sylvian fissures may lose their symmetry

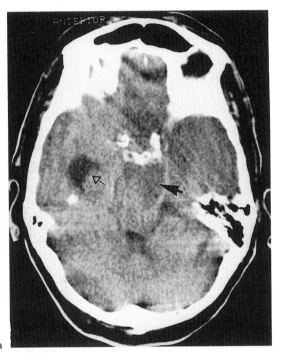

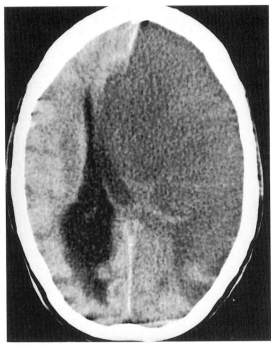

Fig. 5.27 a & b
Massive acute non-haemorrhagic infarct involving ACA and MCA. (a) Uncal herniation with oedematous uncus (arrow) forced through tentorial hiatus. The contralateral temporal horn is obstructed (open arrow). (b) At a more superior level, the swollen, featureless hemisphere is seen. The PCA territory is spared at this stage. The sulci are effaced and there is massive midline shift which is a sign of poor prognosis in this context. The frontal and occipital horns of the L lateral ventricle are approximated indicating subfalcine herniation, and the contralateral ventricle is obstructed.

with the side feeling the effects of the locally enlarging process being compressed or even obliterated. Vulnerable, relatively isolated parts of the ventricular system such as the curved tip of the temporal horn in the middle cranial fossa may be effaced, or obstructed and incarcerated with local dilatation due to trapped CSF. Such well-circumscribed fluid-containing structures should not be confused with true cysts or cystic components of the space-occupying process itself.

As the demand for space increases in what is an unyielding bony environment, further secondary manifestations occur which may be disastrous in themselves. If only one hemisphere is swollen, its ventricle will be compressed and may eventually be pushed under the falx (Fig. 5.27). Such subfalcine herniation is accompanied by an approximation of the frontal and occipital horns of the involved ventricle. If the subfalcine herniation is sufficiently severe, the contralateral ventricle will become obstructed with further local periventricular oedema adding to the rise in intracranial pressure. Nearby vessels or cranial nerves may be trapped against rigid structures such as the edge of the falx or tentorium, or the bony margins of one of the intracranial compartments, with either cata-

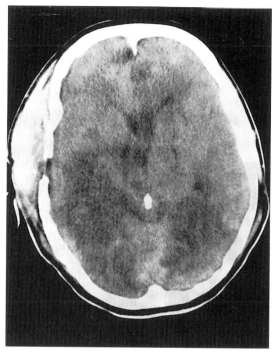

Fig. 5.28
This patient suffered a head injury for which a R craniotomy was required. The degree of brain swelling was unfortunately so severe that the PCAs were trapped, causing extensive secondary infarction in their distribution.

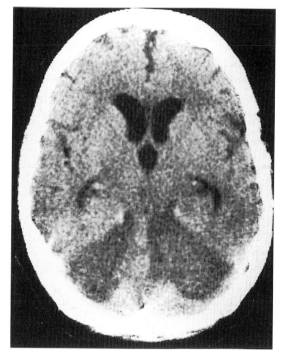

Fig. 5.29
Bilateral acute non-haemorrhagic cerebellar infarcts. The normal crescentic quadrigeminal plate cistern has been completely effaced. The patient died of brain stem compression.

strophic infarction or the production of neurological deficits which are falsely localizing, drawing attention away from the primary pathology (Fig. 5.28). The anterior cerebral artery is particularly vulnerable in cases of subfalcine herniation.

With time, portions of the brain itself will be pushed ahead of a relentlessly advancing process demanding space. The uncus will herniate through the tentorial hiatus (Fig. 5.27) with compromise of the PCA and, finally, contents of the posterior fossa will be forced through the foramen magnum, or superiorly through the tentorium, depending on the direction of the pressure or growth vector.

Brain stem compression ensues, with compromise of vital structures, and death.

Because of the presence of the vulnerable pons and medulla in the posterior fossa, the relatively small proportion of this compartment occupied by compressible ventricle, and the rigid walls of the posterior fossa, decompression craniotomies are commonly performed for space-occupying processes in the posterior fossa regardless of their aetiology (Fig. 5.29).

In the supratentorial compartment, however, particularly if there are large, relatively yielding ventricles, or pre-existing atrophy, a space-occupying process may initially be

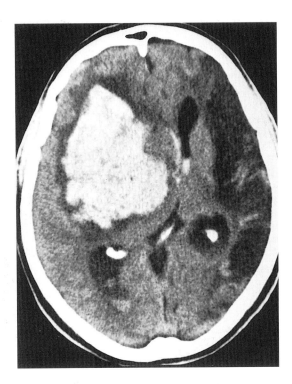

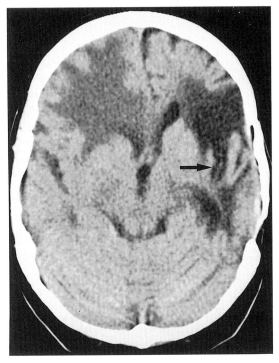

Fig. 5.30
Acute hypertensive haemorrhage in patient with previous gliotic L MCA infarct. A small amount of blood is layering in the R occipital horn. The L lateral ventricle is not showing periventricular oedema at this stage, because of the cushioning effect of the old infarct.

Fig. 5.31
Plain scan showing a mixture of space-creating and space-occupying pathology. There has been an old L craniotomy for meningioma, with dilatation ex vacuo of the L frontal horn and Sylvian fissure (arrow) in which MCA branches can be seen. The gliosis is profoundly low in density. On the R a new tumour is developing, with mass effect shown by the effacement of frontal sulci and compression of the R frontal horn. There is finger-like vasogenic oedema which is appreciably higher in density than the gliosis on the contralateral side.

accommodated more tolerantly. Younger brains with higher turgor are less forgiving. Focal pre-existing atrophic changes will influence the rate of development of symptoms due to a space-occupying process (Fig. 5.30). The shape that this process is allowed to assume will be influenced as well by the local resistance it meets. This is consistent with the basic tenets of military/political theory.

With occasional exceptions such as herpetic encephalitis and other unusual focal inflammatory processes, focal intra-axial space-occupying lesions are nearly always either neoplastic or vascular. Consequently,

the shape of the lesion becomes vital and is discussed below.

Important distinctions between acute vascular and neoplastic processes are summarized at the end of the chapter when their other characteristics have been addressed.

Mixed lesions

Mixed patterns of space creation and space occupation occur. This may be due to related or unrelated pathologies. A brain with

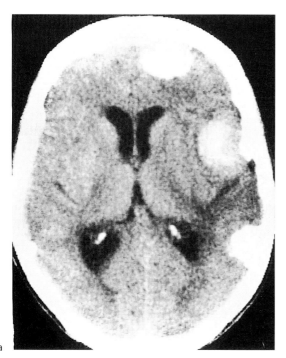
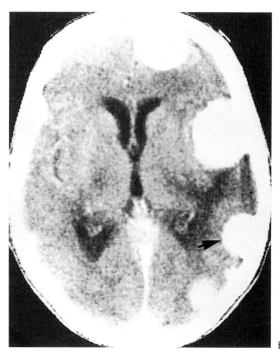

a

b

Fig. 5.32 a & b
Plain (a) and enhanced (b) scans in a patient with multiple meningiomas, clustered over the L hemisphere.
Some of the lesions are hyperdense on the plain scan, due to the presence of calcium. Striking enhancement is seen
after IV contrast, and the number of lesions detectable is increased. The lesion marked with an arrow has been cut
through its epicentre and shows a typical D-shape. The extra-axial location excludes these as metastases, for practical
purposes, and the enhancement pattern excludes them as osteomas. The patient was elderly and had surprisingly few
symptoms.

established atrophy will sometimes have to
accommodate a new space-occupying process
such as a tumour or haemorrhage (Figs 5.30,
5.31). Commonly, however, the mixed
appearance is due to manifestations of the
same pathology in different episodes over
time. The natural history of entities such as
cerebrovascular disease may produce several
episodes of haemorrhage or infarction, and
predisposes to the coincident presence of old
scarring and fresh swelling. Other conditions
which have remitting and relapsing courses
include demyelination due to multiple sclerosis, where an occasional large tumefactive
plaque with mass effect may appear against a

background of multiple atrophic, burned-out
lesions.

Lesions which are unexpectedly space
neutral for their size include progressive multifocal leukoencephalopathy and other white
matter disorders, and some congenital vascular malformations.

Single vs. multiple lesions

Multiple, focal, space-occupying extra-axial
lesions commonly represent benign neoplasms, such as the bilateral acoustic
Schwannomas of Type II neurofibromatosis.
Meningiomas too, are frequently multiple

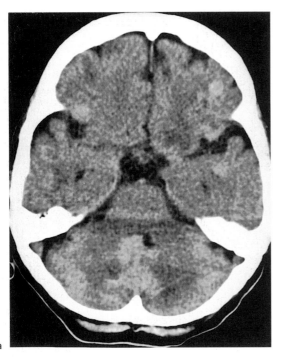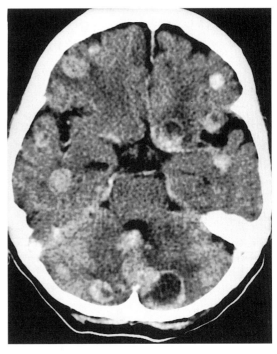

a

b

Fig. 5.33 a & b
Plain (a) and enhanced (b) scans of a patient with multiple intracerebral metastases from a small cell carcinoma of the lung. The IV contrast increases the number and conspicuity of the lesions but in this case the diagnosis could have been made from the plain scan.

and have a combination of physical characteristics allowing quite confident pathological predictions from the image (Fig. 5.32).

Intra-axial lesions have more sinister implications.

If a space-occupying, focal intra-axial lesion is demonstrated and tumour is suspected, important management issues are raised if the lesion is single, or if further similar lesions can be shown. The physical appearances of primary and secondary brain tumours overlap considerably and may be insufficient for a precise diagnosis. The tendency for occasional gliomas to be multifocal also raises some difficulties. If, however, entirely separate similar lesions are identified, the possibility of metastatic dis-

ease becomes much higher. Intravenous contrast agents are often valuable here in showing up additional subtle lesions which may not have been detected on the unenhanced scan. The difference between two and four lesions may be academic (Fig. 5.33), but the difference between one and two is often critical.

Conversely there is major prognostic importance if a solitary lesion is metastatic rather than primary. Overall, some 30% of intracranial metastases are solitary, but the figure rises to 50% for squamous cell carcinoma of the lung. An intracranial lesion is the presenting symptom of a remote malignancy in a significant number of cases. Tumours of the breast, lung and kidney, and

Table 5.10
Multifocal white matter disease

Dysmyelinating
    Multiple hereditary diseases usually presenting
        in childhood
Demyelinating
    Associated with swelling
        Acute disseminated encephalomyelitis
            (auto-immune)
        Tumefactive multiple sclerosis
    Volume neutral (initially)
        Multiple sclerosis
        Progressive multifocal leukoencephalopathy
            (PML)
        Disseminated necrotizing leukoencephalopathy
            associated with chemotherapy and/or
            radiotherapy
    Associated with atrophy
        Age-related leukoencephalopathy
        Chronic stage of any of the above

melanoma cause the majority of intracranial metastases, and attention may be diverted to a likely primary source before surgical intervention in the brain is undertaken.

What suggests that a solitary lesion is metastatic? The presence of a large amount of oedema around a relatively small lesion is useful though not invariable. Location in the posterior fossa in an adult should always suggest metastatic rather than primary disease.

If the metastasis is hyperdense on the plain scan, possibly due to fine particulate calcium, the degree of enhancement which occurs with intravenous contrast is not as striking as, for example, with a meningioma.

Metastatic lesions have a predilection for the grey–white junction but also have a potential for entirely random distribution. When multiple focal abnormalities are seen confined to the white matter, however, a different set of diagnostic possibilities is presented (Table 5.10). Combining the parameters of location, space creation or space occupation and multiplicity helps refine the diagnostic possibilities (Fig. 5.34).

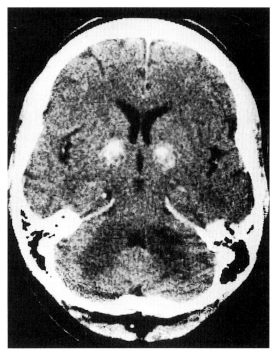

Fig. 5.34
Enhanced scan showing bilateral, volume neutral white matter lesions in the cerebellum (arrows).
Biopsy confirmed progressive multifocal leukoencephalopathy. The symmetry is unusual but not unknown. Incidental basal ganglion calcification is seen.

Physical characteristics of the lesion

Having addressed location, space occupation or creation and number, an individual lesion should be assessed for the following characteristics and properties:

1. Margin
2. Shape
3. Composition
4. Nature of associated oedema
5. Response to intravenous contrast.

Margin
Sharp or straight margins should always raise

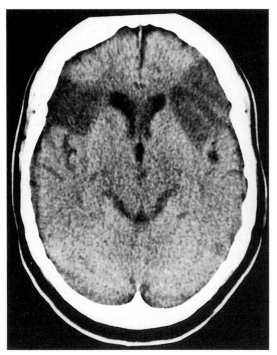

Fig. 5.35
Bilateral symmetrical non-haemorrhagic infarcts involving the superior division of the superficial branches of the middle cerebral arteries. On the L, this includes Broca's speech area. The lesions are sharply demarcated and involve grey and white matter.

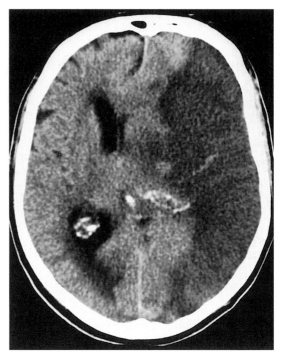

Fig. 5.36
Massive acute L MCA infarct with severe hemispheric swelling and mass effect. Deep and superficial branches are involved. The anterior triangle of frontal lobe supplied by the ACA is spared, as is the head of the caudate nucleus (arrow) which is supplied by the artery of Heubner arising as a recurrent branch of the ACA. The triangle medial to the occipital horn on the left is supplied by the PCA and is also spared.

the possibility of an extra-axial lesion. Intra-axial lesions tend to be less well defined, with the exception of infarcts. Lesions with poorly defined margins suggest infiltration, which correlates with relatively aggressive neo-plasms or spreading infections.

PML has a characteristically scalloped margin which distinguishes it from other white matter lesions.

A margin may sharpen with time, as with an evolving infarct or inflammatory lesion with remission of oedema, and with healing processes that more clearly define the boundaries between normal and abnormal tissue.

Shape
It is essential to look at all the slices which contain the lesion to obtain a 3-dimensional grasp of its shape. Tumours are generally round with occasional specific morphology such as a dumb-bell shape dictated by the presence of a bony barrier such as may be seen with Schwannomas at the petrous apex. Durally-based lesions such as meningiomas classically have a D-shape.

Lesions where shape is particularly useful in diagnosis are dominated by the group containing infarcts (Figs 5.35, 5.36, 5.37).

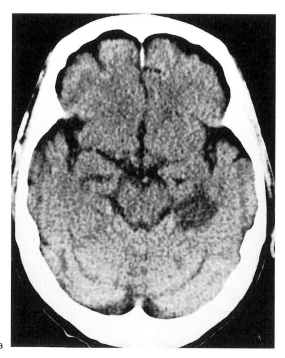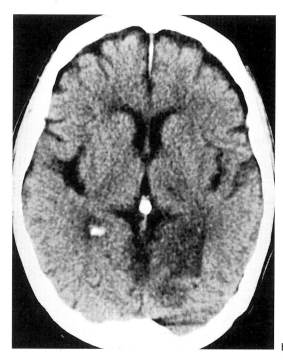

a   b

Fig. 5.37 a & b
a & b (Unenhanced scans)
Posterior cerebral artery territory infarction.
(a) Hypodense infarct on the undersurface of the temporal lobe. Note its medial limitation by the faintly visible edge of the tentorium. If seen in isolation, the ischaemic basis of this lesion may not be immediately apparent.
(b) More superiorly, the same patient shows more characteristic features of a PCA infarct involving the occipital lobe.

Infarcts are geometric, but may be incomplete depending on the severity and extent of tissue damage and the availability of collaterals. At mid-ventricular level, extrapolation of straight lines from the frontal and occipital horns to the calvarium defines the triangular territories of the anterior cerebral artery (ACA) and posterior cerebral artery (PCA) and quadrilateral or trapezoidal middle cerebral artery (MCA) territories (Fig. 3.21).

The shapes of the vascular territories change radically once one departs from this mid-ventricular level, but there are still a few lesions which from their shape and location may readily be recognized as vascular, particularly if they are in continuity with other ischaemic lesions in the same territory. An example is the 'strip' lesion on the undersurface of the temporal lobe which indicates a PCA lesion. Another characteristically shaped lesion is the scythe-shaped posterior inferior cerebellar artery (PICA) infarct, which is the commonest infarct seen in young adults. This parallels the inner table in a curve and extends sagittally towards V4.

Brain stem infarcts pose a special challenge. Large lesions are seldom seen on CT because the damage to vital structures precludes survival. Smaller lesions provoke relatively little oedema or density change, and their identification may be hampered by the interpetrous artefact. In the midbrain, the lesions may be midline, but in the pons and medulla they tend to be unilateral, paramedian and sharply defined medially, with their long axes in the sagittal plane. This reflects the distribution of the penetrating arteries. Lateral infarcts are less common and are due to lesions in the short circumferential vessels.

The shape of a vascular lesion may be less than classical, if the entire territory has not been involved. Commonly only the central part of the artery's distribution will be affected, with collaterals maintaining perfusion to the periphery. The extent of the vascular insult depends on the rapidity of the vessel occlusion (embolus versus thrombosis), the perfusion pressure, the condition of the artery prior to the event, and the availability of collaterals.

Of all vessels, the middle cerebral artery (MCA) is most commonly involved with thrombosis, embolism and haemorrhage. It carries the largest proportion of intracerebral blood flow and has a long course. Its peripheral branches are relatively far away from the brain base collaterals. The penetrating branches are subject to high arterial pressures and are consequently vulnerable. Familiarity with its distribution is therefore essential.

Combinations of lesions in vessel territories have clinical significance. Lesions in both ACA and MCA may point to an abnormality in the carotid itself, such as a dissection. Combinations of MCA and PCA lesions suggest good flow connections between anterior and posterior circulations on that side through the circle of Willis, or else two different lesions. Lesions in opposite hemispheres, especially in a young patient, raise the possibility of an extracranial abnormality such as a cardiac source for emboli.

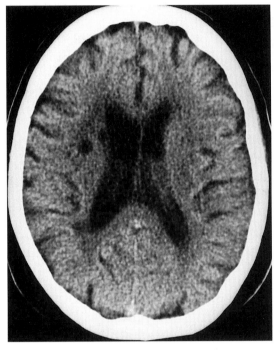

Fig. 5.38
Two small lacunar infarcts adjacent to the R lateral ventricle.

Angulation of the slice may introduce an elongation distortion and this must be recognized in the assessment of both the location and shape of a lesion. For example, scanning parallel to the skull base projects the central sulcus of the cortex quite posteriorly, and also projects the furthest limit of the strip of ACA supply in its paramedian location at the vertex quite posteriorly.

Other curved processes include extracerebral collections, dealt with in detail later. Subdurals are the commonest, and spread in an extensive but shallow fashion over the brain surface and are thus C-shaped. Occasionally, loculations in the posterior interhemispheric fissure, as seen in non-accidental paediatric injury, or spreading

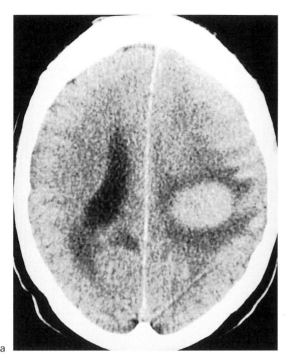 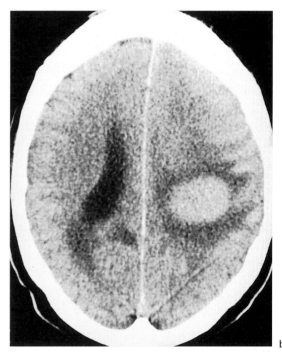

a   b

Fig. 5.39 a & b
(a) Plain and (b) enhanced scans showing a focus of intracerebral NHL. The lesion is hyperdense and diffusely enhancing, and surrounded by vasogenic oedema.

over the tentorial surface, will produce a relatively pancake-shaped lesion. Extradurals on the other hand tend to be elliptical.

Small distinctively shaped intra-axial processes include the triangular appearance of central pontine myelinolysis (Fig. 5.23) and the round to oval contour of lacunar infarction (Fig. 5.38).

Tubular or fusiform shapes should suggest a blood vessel abnormality. In isolation centrally in the brainstem, syringobulbia must be considered.

Composition
• *Solid*
Solid lesions may be homogeneous or heterogeneous. Homogeneous lesions imply a more orderly growth pattern and often a reasonable prognosis, and heterogeneous lesions a disorderly process, though exceptions such as teratomas do occur. Ependymomas are characteristically heterogeneous compared with medulloblastomas. Lymphomas are commonly uniform in density (Fig. 5.39), while the least differentiated, highest grade gliomas (glioblastoma multiforme) often have central necrosis contributing to a bizarre appearance (Fig. 5.40).

On the unenhanced scan a lesion may be described as hypodense (Fig. 5.41), isodense or hyperdense to surrounding brain, and this too has diagnostic implications (Tables 5.11, 5.12). The majority of focal intracranial lesions, including tumours, are hypodense to

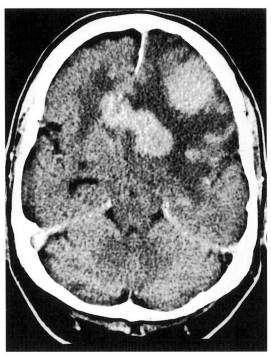

Fig. 5.40
Enhanced scan of a grade IV astrocytoma (glioblastoma) with heterogeneous appearance, transcallosal spread and marked local mass effect.

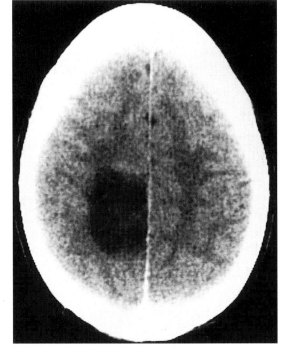

Fig. 5.41
Plain scan showing reasonably well circumscribed hypodense ganglioglioma. A low grade astrocytoma could be similar in appearance.

Table 5.11
Hypodense lesions (pre-contrast)

Neoplasms
  Gliomas
  Ganglioglioma
  Fat-containing lesions including lipomas, dermoids
  Colloid cysts (variable)
  Metastases especially from epithelial tumours
Damaged brain
  Infarction without macroscopic haemorrhage
  Necrosis of globus pallidus associated with hypoxia, hypotension, hypoglycaemia, carbon monoxide and barbiturate poisoning, etc.
  Radiation necrosis
  Resolving haematoma
Inflammatory/infective lesions
  Focal encephalitis e.g. herpes
  Cerebritis
  Tumefactive demyelination

Table 5.12
Hyperdense lesions (pre-contrast)

Neoplasms
  Meningioma
  Lymphoma
  Medulloblastoma
  Metastatic disease esp. from tumours with dense cellular structure, osteoid or calcification, and vascular tumours such as choriocarcinoma and melanoma
Developmental
  Arteriovenous malformations, cavernomas
Acute haemorrhage
Dystrophically calcified lesions

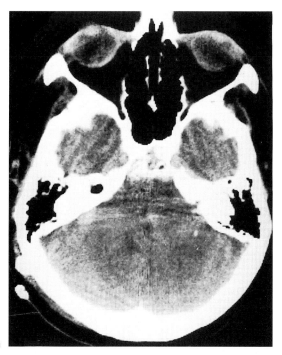
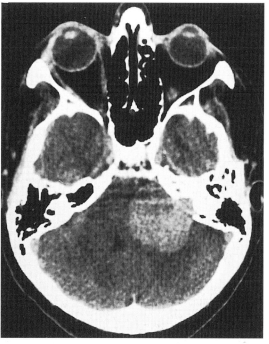

a

b

Fig. 5.42 a & b
(a) Plain and (b) enhanced scans of a large L acoustic Schwannoma. On the plain study the isodense tumour is difficult to see, and this is compounded by the interpetrous artefact. The displaced fourth ventricle gives the clue. The enhanced scan shows the lesion and also the destruction of the posterior IAC wall.

brain, so the hyperdense group have particular diagnostic significance. The isodense lesions pose the greatest perceptual difficulties, especially if they are too small to produce mass effect. Chief among these are the acoustic Schwannoma (Fig. 5.42), and those very well-differentiated fibrillary astrocytomas which most closely mimic normal brain.

• *Cystic*
Cystic lesions must be distinguished from low density and necrotic lesions, and this is not always easy. The most reliable way to identify a cystic lesion is to see a fluid–fluid (Fig. 5.43) or air–fluid level. The density of the fluid content may be similar to or higher

than CSF (Fig. 5.44). The presence of an enhancing mural nodule in a cystic mass raises the strong possibility of haemangioblastoma if the lesion is found in the posterior fossa of a young woman (Fig. 5.45).

• *Fat-containing*
Lipomas (Fig. 5.46) occur as small isolated tumours commonly in the ventricles, interhemispheric fissure, quadrigeminal plate cistern, or in association with partial AGCC. Fat may also be seen in dermoids and teratomas, but not usually in epidermoids where the cholesterol present is in a solid rather than a liquid state. The density of fat is lower than CSF, and in the negative Hu range (-70 to -100), but not as low as air.

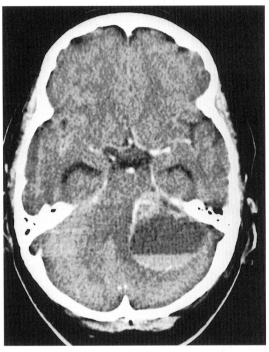

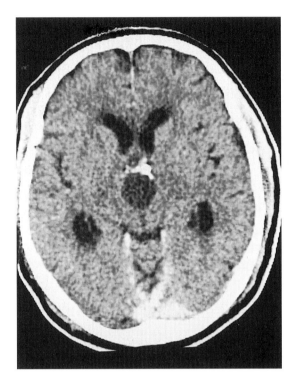

Fig. 5.43   (*above left*)
Enhanced scan showing fluid–fluid level due to haemorrhage into a cyst associated with an acoustic Schwannoma. The patient was having a new breast cancer staged, and the importance of excluding this mass as metastatic was paramount. There was no oedema, and further slices showed the lesion to be extra-axial.

Fig. 5.44   (*above right*)
Intraventricular glioma with cyst formation and calcium. The density is slightly higher than CSF, and the mass should not be mistaken for a distended third ventricle.

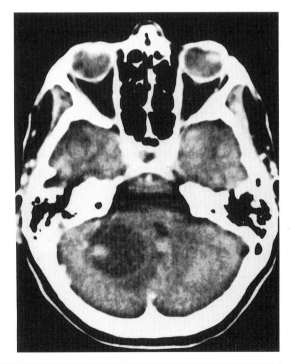

Fig. 5.45   (*right*)
Cerebellar haemangioblastoma.

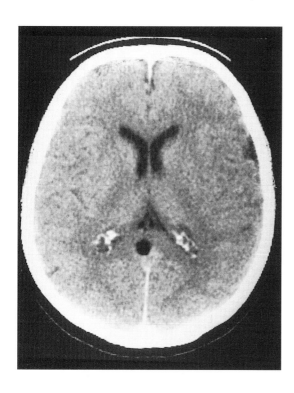

Fig. 5.46 (*left*)
Quadrigeminal plate cistern lipoma.

Fig. 5.47 a & b (*below*)
Amyloid angiopathy producing intraparenchymal haemorrhage. (a) L frontal haematoma with mass effect. (b) 1 year later, a fresh R frontal haematoma is seen. Signs of focal atrophy have developed on the L.

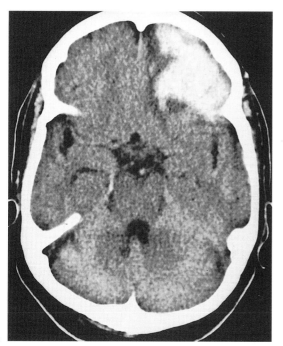

a

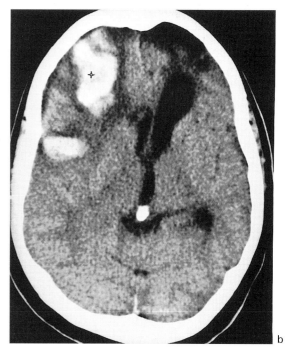

b

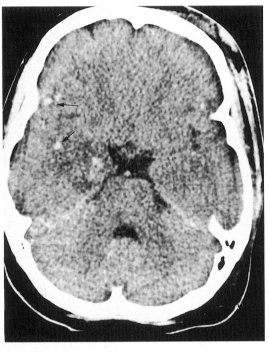

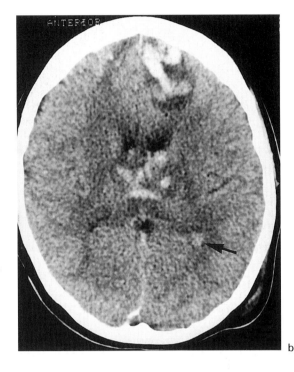

a

b

Fig. 5.48 a & b
Trauma. (a) Small petechial haemorrhages (arrows) raising the possibility of a shearing injury. (b) More confluent contusions and bleeding in L frontal and callosal regions. Blood is present in the L trigone (arrow).

Table 5.13
Major causes of multiple intracranial haemorrhage

Trauma
Shearing injuries with petechial haemorrhage
Contusions
Vascular
Multiple haemorrhagic infarcts
 – if arterial, suspect emboli
 – if venous, suspect deep venous or sinus
  thrombosis
Amyloid angiopathy
Vasculitis e.g. SLE
Neoplastic
Vascular metastatic lesions notably melanoma,
 renal carcinoma, choriocarcinoma
Systemic
Hypertensive haemorrhage
Anticoagulation

Table 5.14
Multiple intracranial calcifications

Physiologic
Pineal, habenula, choroid, dura, vascular, basal
 ganglia, petroclinoid ligament
Post infective/inflammatory
Viral, parasitic and protozoal infections
 especially cysticercosis and the childhood
 TORCH syndromes
Neoplastic
Multiple benign neoplasms
Metastatic deposits
Syndrome related
Tuberous sclerosis
Sturge–Weber syndrome(encephalotrigeminal
 angiomatosis)
von Hippel–Lindau (cerebro-retinal
 angiomatosis)
Other dystrophic deposits
Damaged tissue from multiple causes including
 trauma, ischaemia, radiation
Metabolic
Disturbances of calcium and phosphate
 metabolism

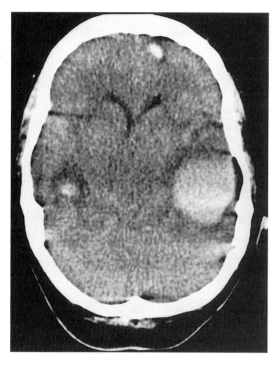

Fig. 5.49
Plain scan showing haemorrhage into multiple melanomatous deposits. Both focal and global swelling are present.

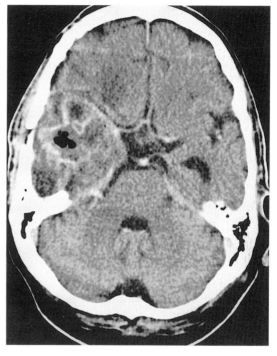

Fig. 5.50
Ring-enhancing R temporal lobe abscess following craniotomy.

• *Blood*

Focal intraparenchymal haemorrhage (Fig. 5.30) is most commonly associated with a hypertensive rupture of a degenerative Charcot–Bouchard aneurysm on one of the penetrating arteries, or with an underlying vascular malformation, though as hypertension and other population risk factors are being controlled, amyloid (congophilic) angiopathic haemorrhage is assuming greater importance (Fig. 5.47). Causes of multiple haemorrhages are shown in Table 5.13 (Figs 5.48, 5.49) and the physical evolution of haemorrhage over time will be discussed later.

• *Air*

Air is rarely seen within cerebral abscesses unless there has been trauma or surgery (Fig. 5.50). Bubbles of air are more suspicious of infection than long air–fluid levels which may persist for days to weeks after surgery. Intraventricular or extracerebral air (pneumocephalus) in the setting of trauma implies a compound fracture or involvement of an aerated sinus.

• *Calcium*

Causes of multiple intracranial calcifications are shown in Table 5.14, and neoplasms which calcify in Table 5.15.

Table 5.15
Calcifying intracranial neoplasms

Gliomas
  Oligodendrogliomas (commonly)
  Low grade astrocytomas
Meningiomas
Craniopharyngiomas
  Especially paediatric type
Metastatic
  Osteocartilaginous tumours including
    osteosarcomas
  Mucin-secreting adenocarcinomas of colon and
    ovary
Benign lesions
  Angioma, hamartoma, neurofibroma
Other
  Lipoma of corpus callosum
  Choroid plexus papilloma
  Ependymoma

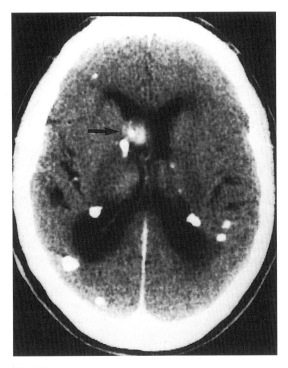

Fig. 5.51
Calcification in tuberous sclerosis. A giant cell astrocytoma is developing at the typical location, close to the foramen of Monro (arrow). These lesions normally enhance strongly.

Normal calcification
The pineal, habenular and choroid plexuses normally accumulate calcium as the patient ages. In people over middle age, calcium is frequently detected in the major intracranial arteries, and scattered through the lentiform nuclei.

Abnormal calcification
Here the calcium deposition is regarded as abnormal, regardless of the patient's age. It falls into 3 broad categories.

Local/specific
Certain tumours are prone to produce calcium as a useful distinguishing feature. The calcium associated with oligodendrogliomas is coarse and craggy and helps to differentiate this tumour from other primary glial lesions. Meningiomas also calcify with increasing maturity. Certain metastatic lesions such as mucin-secreting adenocarcinomas or osteosarcomas also contain calcium and can help direct the search for the primary site.

Congenital lesions with a vascular basis such as Sturge–Weber syndrome or arteriovenous malformations may also show characteristic calcification which is usually linear or serpiginous.

Dystrophic
This is the commonest cause of intracranial calcification and reflects the predilection of calcium for deposition in areas of old inflammation, trauma, infarction or other causes of damaged or abnormal brain. It is commonly part of a healing process in the chronic stage. Examples include granulomas, old subdural collections and areas

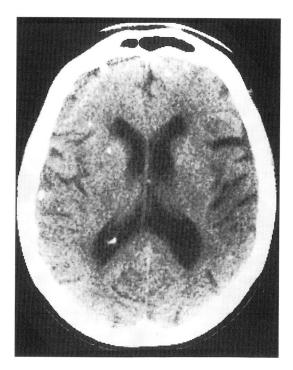

Fig. 5.52
Dystrophic calcification in cysticercosis. The patient had acquired epilepsy.

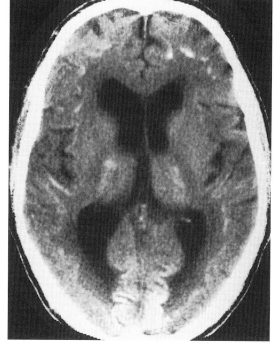

Fig. 5.53
Metastatic calcification in the occipital cortex and diffusely through the grey–white junction, in a patient with chronic renal failure.

of gliosis resulting from a range of insults (Figs 5.51, 5.52).

Metastatic

Here the pathology is systemic, and reflects a high circulating level of blood calcium commonly associated with parathyroid disorders or other metabolic conditions including chronic lead exposure. Calcium may be deposited anywhere, but the grey–white junction is a favoured location (Fig. 5.53).

- *Differentiation of calcium from blood*

Unusually heavy basal ganglion calcification or other dense focal deposits have occasionally been mistaken for areas of fresh haemorrhage. Attention to the Hounsfield numbers will resolve such cases, with calcific deposits reading significantly higher than the 80–100 Hu of fresh blood. The actual reading depends on the density of the calcium deposit but is commonly well in excess of 100 Hu. Even to the naked eye, however, there is a difference: fresh blood has a softer, fluffier look, and will exert mass effect proportional to its size and the degree of oedema present. Calcium has a hard, bright and brittle look, and when associated with a dystrophic process may be accompanied by local atrophy, depending on the aetiology. The clinical history is of course essential, as the presence of fresh haemorrhage is usually accompanied by an acute neurological deficit.

Oedema

There are 3 major types of oedema: periventricular, vasogenic and cytotoxic, which may occur in combination but reflect different pathophysiology.

Periventricular (interstitial) oedema

This is caused by fluid stasis in the tissues close to the ventricular ependyma, and reflects an active disturbance in CSF transport dynamics. This observation is more useful than simple assessment of ventricular size. The oedema begins at the angles of the frontal and occipital horns and is hazy and indistinct (Fig. 5.1), which is valuable in the distinction from periventricular gliosis (Fig. 5.2).

Vasogenic oedema

This is a recognizable and ominous form of oedema, associated with abnormal leakage of proteinaceous fluid from damaged cells into the extracellular space. The fluid spreads readily through the white matter, dropping its density, exaggerating its contrast against grey matter and producing a margin with characteristic finger-like projections. Mass effect is inevitable and proportional to the amount of oedema fluid, a useful distinguishing feature from other low-density white matter pathology (Fig. 5.54).

With increasing severity there will be compression effects on adjacent grey matter structures, but the white matter emphasis remains discernible until late.

Vasogenic oedema is a sinister finding, suggesting tumour, inflammation or another cause of BBB breakdown. It is not normally associated with infarcts. It should be investigated until a cause is found. It also has management implications as it responds, at least initially, to steroid therapy and may temporarily ameliorate the symptoms of a patient with an intra-axial neoplasm. The nature of the underlying process, however, often remains sinister and ultimately governs prognosis.

Cytotoxic oedema

This implies the swelling of cells, both in grey and white matter, frequently in response to a metabolic disturbance such as ischaemia, which causes failure of the sodium/potassium pump. Grey–white differentiation is lost, rather than exaggerated, because grey matter with its higher basal metabolic rate is more vulnerable and swells more, dropping its Hu towards that of white matter.

Cytotoxic oedema may be diffuse (Table 5.5) or focal. The commonest cause of the focal form is cerebral ischaemia, where all the tissues in the path of a stricken vessel are affected. Infarcts thus characteristically involve both grey and white matter, though in very young children the relatively high metabolic demands of the myelinating white matter make it more vulnerable. In adults the cortical grey matter has a far higher metabolic rate, accounting for the high incidence of cortical involvement in focal ischaemia. Damage following ischaemia may not be permanent, with a variable amount of tissue at the periphery obtaining sufficient perfusion from collaterals to recover and regain normal density. The extent and rapidity of the development of the oedema correlates with lesion severity. If perfusion is not re-established, permanent damage occurs, with cell death, myelin breakdown and gliosis or myelomalacia over time.

Pattern recognition here relies on the identification of involvement of a particular vessel territory.

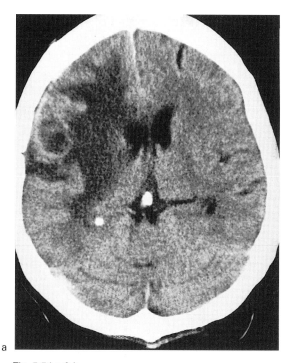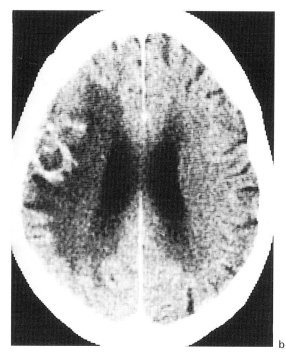

a   b

Fig. 5.54 a & b
(a) Enhanced scan showing peripheral ring-enhancing tumour with extensive vasogenic oedema, straddling vascular territories and predominantly, but not exclusively, involving white matter. Sulcal effacement and frontal horn deformity testify to the mass effect.
(b) Same patient scanned elsewhere 14 weeks later, after radiotherapy. The ring-enhancing tumour is still present, but the white matter changes, despite being more extensive, are not showing mass effect, as they are due in part to ischaemic damage induced by radiotherapy. Acute focal radionecrosis can show mass effect. Radiotherapy may produce a gradual endarteritis with worsening of the patient's clinical condition and deterioration in global cerebral function.

Response to intravenous contrast

This can provide additional useful discriminating information if approached along the following lines:

- Does the lesion enhance or not?
- How quickly does it blush and how long does the effect last?
- Is there a particular pattern to the enhancement i.e. ring, serpiginous, diffuse or patchy?
- Is this enhancement part of an evolving process?

In order to pose these questions, one needs an understanding of the common mechanisms of enhancement with iodinated agents in the head.

Mechanisms of enhancement
- *Vascular lesions*
Truly vascular lesions, such as arteriovenous malformations (AVMs) and venous angiomas, will reflect their vascular nature when the Hounsfield number of the blood is raised by the administration of iodinated material (Figs 5.55, 5.56, 5.57). The more profuse

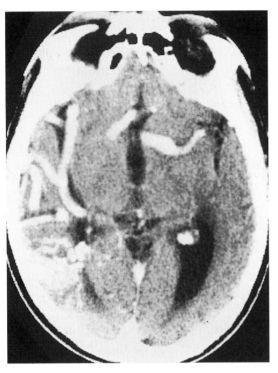

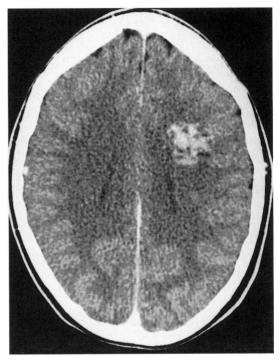

Fig. 5.55 +C
**Opacification of blood within the channels of a large
AVM.** The hypertrophied vessels of the circle of Willis are
evident, and could be seen on the plain scan, as could
the congenital disorganization of the grey and white
matter in the R parietal region. This elderly patient had
epilepsy following partial infarction of the lesion.

Fig. 5.56 +C
**Angiographically occult vascular malformation
(AOVM) which was hyperdense on plain scan and
enhanced in a mild, diffuse manner.** The patient
presented in his late teens with epilepsy.

the arterial supply is, the more rapidly and
readily this will be observed. A crude angio-
graphic-type profile of the rate of change of
the Hounsfield values of individual lesions is
obtainable with some machines and can give
an idea of the flow kinetics or how rapidly a
lesion is being perfused with opacified blood.
The effect will fade rapidly as the contrast
agent is filtered into the extravascular space
which will occur wherever there is no blood–
brain barrier to prevent it. Enhancement
remains noticeable in the head longer than in
the body, especially if narrow window photo-

graphic techniques are used which will
emphasize subtle persisting density changes.

Lesions with a rich blood supply, such as
vascular meningiomas, will also owe part of
their enhancement to this, though other factors such as a lack of blood–brain barrier will
be operating.

● *Absent blood–brain barrier (BBB)*
Extra-axial structures by definition lack a
BBB, and normally enhance. These include
the anterior pituitary and the meninges, and
tumours of extra-axial origin.

Generally the most de-differentiated tumours will have the most poorly developed blood–brain barriers and will show the most enhancement, as is seen with the high grade gliomas. Eventually necrosis will occur in rapidly growing tumours and those necrotic areas will lose their ability to enhance.

● *Collaterals and neovascularity*

The use of intravenous contrast agents in the setting of clinically obvious acute ischaemia has declined. One reason is that most of the mechanisms responsible for post-ischaemic enhancement are not operable within the first days to a week after the event. After this, neovascularity develops to complement collateral flow, producing so-called luxury perfusion with visible enhancement. By 2 to 3 weeks, however, when useful enhancement should have developed, the diagnosis is seldom in doubt.

● *Other factors*

Other factors such as myelin breakdown undoubtedly operate in producing abnormal enhancement in the brain, but their mechanisms are not well understood.

The observation of enhancement may therefore be useful, but failure to observe enhancement may relate to many factors. They range from the origin, development and differentiation of the tissue in question, to the timing in the natural history of the process. Early in ischaemia and inflammation no enhancement may be seen, but this may be visible later as the mechanisms described above have time to show their effects. Often more than one mechanism will be at work at any one time, though their effects will overlap. Blood–brain barrier breakdown, for example, will declare itself before the manifestations of neovascularity.

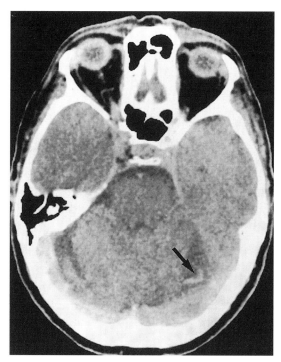

Fig. 5.57   +C
Small cerebellar venous angioma (arrow) with local atrophy presumably due to stealing. Vascular malformations may show mild mass effect, be volume neutral or cause atrophy, as here.

● *Damaged or defective BBB*

Many factors can damage the normal blood–brain barrier, ranging from trauma and infection to ischaemia and radiation. The effect may be temporary, as in epilepsy, and only last a few hours, or it may persist and be overtaken by reparative processes, as in the case of evolving infarcts. Usually it lasts from weeks to months and is altered by healing or scarring processes which are taking place at the same time.

Tumours which do not have or which by de-differentiation have lost their similarity to normal brain tissue will also enhance.

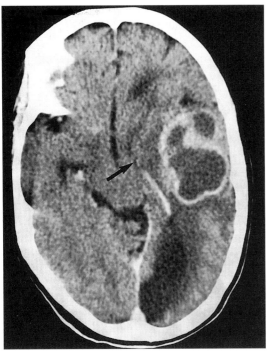

Fig. 5.58   +C
High grade glioma showing ring enhancement and impending uncal herniation (arrow). The PCA has been trapped against the tent causing an occipital infarct.

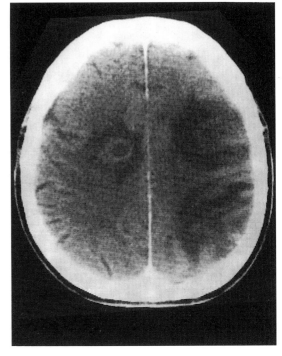

Fig. 5.59   +C
Ring enhancement of toxoplasmosis in patient with AIDS. The ring is thinner medially which is a feature of abscesses. Further lesions are in evolution on the L.

Table 5.16
Ring-enhancing lesions

Neoplastic
  High grade gliomas
  Metastases
  Lymphoma
Infective
  Abscesses
Reparative
  Resolving haematoma or infarct
  Post-irradiation

Patterns of enhancement

- *Ring enhancement*

This is a relatively non-specific appearance (Table 5.16), and most commonly due to resolving vascular lesions or tumours (Fig. 5.58). In an immune-compromised population infection will be higher on the list (Fig. 5.59).

- *Diffuse enhancement*

Solid homogeneous tumours including medulloblastoma and lymphoma will enhance diffusely, as will extra-axial masses. The enhancement is usually mild. If striking, meningioma should be considered.

A patchy variation occurs in heterogeneous lesions.

- *Serpiginous*

This pattern must suggest a vascular lesion (Fig. 5.55).

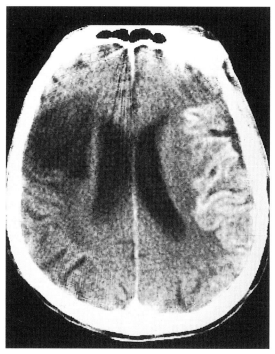

Fig. 5.60   +C
Old and new MCA infarcts. On the R, an old infarct is present, with gliosis close to CSF density, and a dilated lateral ventricle. The L shows diffuse gyral enhancement (toothpaste) in the distribution of the MCA, with mild mass effect on the ventricle.

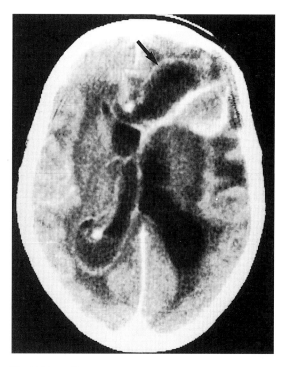

Fig. 5.61   +C
Mixed enhancement pattern. A L frontal haematoma has been evacuated, with intense ring enhancement of the bed aggravated by superadded infection. The L frontal horn is obstructed and infected. The R LV is also infected and shows ependymal enhancement. Dependent debris is present.

● *Gyral*

This is a useful, specific pattern associated with ischaemia or radiation injury. It is a transient phenomenon, and the area of enhancement may exceed the final area of irreversible damage (Fig. 5.60). A rare, persisting cause is superficial angioma formation or neovascularity involving the leptomeninges.

● *Ependymal*

This usually indicates infection (Fig. 5.61) or tumour.

Effects of time

Acute space-occupying processes constitute the greatest neurological challenge to diagnosis and treatment. Knowledge of how a process should behave with time can be useful in identifying it, ageing it and giving prognostic information.

A tumour which has already produced symptoms will, in the absence of treatment, increase in size, with the most aggressive and poorly differentiated lesions showing the most rapid growth. The tumour itself grows,

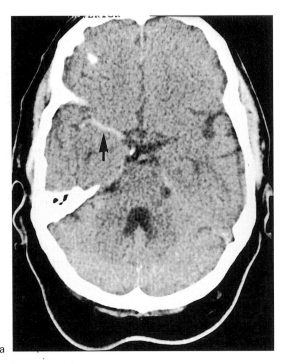
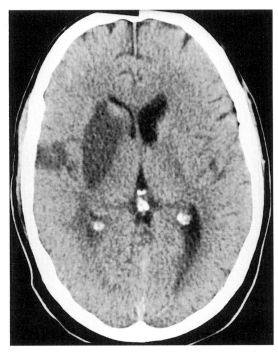

a

b

Fig. 5.62 a & b
(a) Plain scan within 24 hours of acute ischaemia. The only clue to its presence is the hyperdense R MCA (arrow) suspicious of stasis or thrombosis. (b) Three days later, a basal ganglionic and patchy superficial infarct has developed in the R MCA territory, with mass effect.

and the vasogenic oedema it excites also increases relentlessly.

With an ischaemic lesion a certain pre-dictable pattern is seen, if no further insult occurs. Its behaviour with time is one of its most useful diagnostic characteristics.

A scan performed in the first 24 hours after a bland infarct is frequently normal. This has prognostic significance, as more severe infarcts become visible more rapidly. After 24 hours, infarcts show as hypodense areas corresponding to part or the whole of a recognized vessel territory (Fig. 5.62). Over 90% show no macroscopic haemorrhage, though microscopy will reveal petechial haemorrhage and MR studies have confirmed that some cortical bleeding is common.

Generally speaking, a frankly haemorrhagic infarct, especially if in the peripheral MCA territory, raises the possibility of embolic rather than thrombotic disease, because of the abrupt shock to the autoregulatory mech-anisms governing capillary permeability. Any infarct which is sufficiently large can, how-ever, bleed, and patients with impaired coag-ulation are also at risk of secondary haemorrhage into an infarct. The presence of macroscopic blood visible on CT early in the course of an ischaemic event is frequently associated with a more severe deficit.

Nevertheless, it remains true that the vast majority of fresh infarcts are 'bland'. A brief 'fogging' phenomenon has been described a few days after the event if petechial haemor-

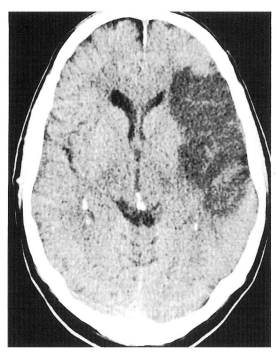 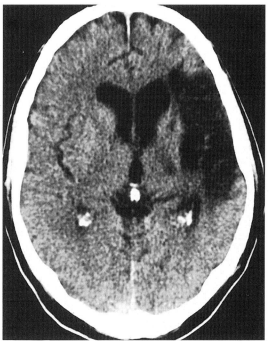

a　　　　　　　　　　　　　　　　　　　　　　　　　　　　　　　　　　　　b

Fig. 5.63 a & b
Plain scans 8 months apart showing the classic evolution of a trapezoidal L MCA infarct. Initially (a) only the superficial branches are involved. The lesion is mildly hypodense; the ventricles are small, and the absence of L frontal sulci is due to swelling transmitted through the L hemisphere. Later (b) the infarct has dropped in density almost to CSF levels. The ventricles have enlarged, particularly the L frontal horn. Lacunar lesions have appeared in the distribution of the thalamostriate perforators.

rhage raises the Hu of the infarct towards that of brain, but this is seldom encountered in practice.

If the clinical course is unexpected or the diagnosis is in doubt, the patient is re-scanned. The typical evolution of a bland infarct is for its mass effect to plateau and then regress visibly after 1 to 2 weeks. The margin of the infarct becomes progressively more sharply demarcated. Enhancement is seldom seen at the time of maximal mass effect, but begins to develop by the end of the first week, and persists with a bell-shaped curve of incidence for up to 3 months. On plain scans, the Hu drops further as neutral

fat released from damaged myelin is phago-cytosed. As gliosis proceeds, a stable low density lesion with local atrophy is usually established by 3 months (Fig. 5.63).

With intracerebral haematomas, a pre-dictable pattern of evolution is also seen. Acutely extravasated blood is seen almost instantly with CT, due to the high Hu of haemoglobin. The narrow window settings normally used show fresh blood as hyper-dense to brain, making it readily visible, irre-spective of the aetiology of the haemorrhage. A halo of oedema develops within 24 hours. If a clot is formed which retracts, the Hu reading may temporarily rise even further. As

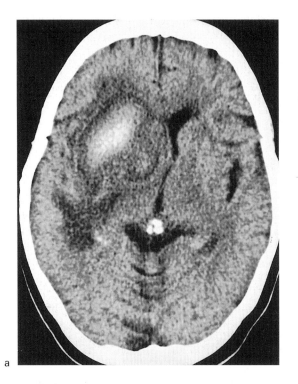

a

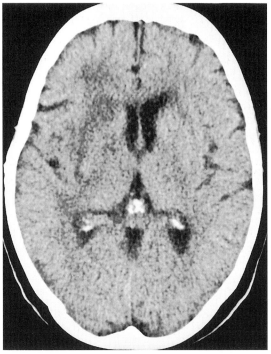

b

Fig. 5.64 a, b & c
(a) −C. Basal ganglionic haematoma at 2 weeks. Hyperdense blood persists, but the margins are becoming fuzzy and indistinct. A halo of oedema contributes to the mass effect. **(b) −C and (c) +C scans 1 month later.** The blood has resorbed leaving a vague hypodense area which shows ring enhancement with IV contrast. The mass effect is resolving slowly, but the appearance could still suggest a tumour if taken in isolation without the serial images.

c

lysis occurs, fluid–fluid levels may occur, especially in hypercoagulable or anaemic states but possible in any large haematoma.

Further episodes of bleeding or oozing may occur, but once the haemodynamics have stabilized, resolution of the haematoma begins slowly, from the outside inwards, with a slow reduction in mass effect as oedema and blood products are resorbed. The margin becomes indistinct (Fig. 5.64) and fades, and visible coalescent haemorrhage is seldom seen beyond 6 weeks, though MRI will show persisting blood breakdown products such as methaemoglobin and haemosiderin for months to years beyond this. The age of a haematoma may therefore often be estimated from its CT appearance. Conversely, if the age appears inappropriate, the clinical situation must be reconsidered.

Time is a powerful and underutilized diagnostic tool.

Effects of gravity

Gravity can produce air–fluid or fluid–fluid levels. An air–fluid level in the sphenoid sinus is an indicator of a possible skull base fracture. Tilting the head slightly will distinguish between a true level and a pseudolevel produced by incomplete pneumatization of the sinus.

In the ventricles, purulent material (Fig. 5.61) or blood will sink to the most dependent parts which are the occipital horns, and these are thus rewarding to inspect in cases of suspected subarachnoid haemorrhage. Tilting will also distinguish these from partial volume artefact.

Haemorrhage into cystic tumours or chronic extracerebral collections can have the different densities of their fluid contents distinguished in this way as well as having

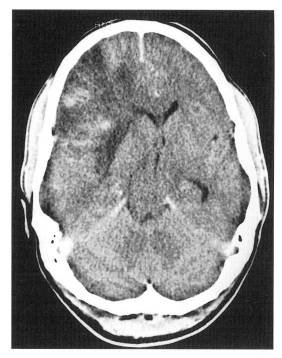

Fig. 5.65   +C
Grade III astrocytoma in young patient. Abrupt onset suggested infarct. The lesion is indeed roughly geometric but clearly straddles MCA and ACA territory. There is sparing of the cortical grey of the R frontal lobe. The enhancement is bizarre and has appeared too soon in the clinical course for an infarct. The lentiform nucleus is presenting a temporary barrier to the spread of vasogenic oedema.

their fluid nature confirmed (Fig. 5.43). The contents may be moved by tilting to distinguish hyperdense material such as blood lying next to another hyperdense structure such as an enhancing wall, or if a nodular excrescence from the wall could be being obscured by blood.

Discrimination between tumour and infarct

Although a wide range of pathology has been covered by this chapter, it is clear in clinical

Table 5.17
Discrimination between intra-axial tumour and infarct

	Tumour	Infarct
Shape	Variable. Irregular or round.	Wedge-shaped with cortical base; quadrilateral/trapezoidal or incomplete manifestations of these.
Margin	Vague, lobulated.	Relatively sharp, straight.
Relation to vascular territory	No obvious relationship. May overlap territories.	Conforms to vessel territory shape or less. Watershed type will straddle adjacent territories.
Oedema pattern	Vasogenic with cortical sparing.	Cytotoxic (grey plus white matter frequently involved).
Enhancement pattern	Enhancement usually present at time of presentation, except for extremely well-differentiated lesions. Pattern may be diffuse, heterogeneous, ring-like or nodular.	Usually no enhancement in first few days after event, and rarely persisting beyond 3 months. When present, may be variable, but gyral pattern characteristic. Enhancement maximal after the period of maximal mass effect.
Mass effect over time	May reduce with steroids – generally relentlessly increasing.	Maximal towards end of first week; then plateaus and progressively reduces if uncomplicated.
Ancillary findings	Other lesions if metastatic (parenchymal, meningeal, calvarial); known syndromes or associations e.g. von Hippel–Lindau.	Evidence of other ischaemic lesions; visible vascular abnormality (stasis, thrombosis, calcification etc).
Clinical caveats	Course may fluctuate with oedema.	Course may be complicated by further infarction, bleeding, extracranial influences e.g. hydration, medication.

practice that a frequently faced dilemma is that of the patient presenting with a solitary acute intra-axial space-occupying process, where the distinction between tumour and infarct must be made (Fig. 5.65). The history is clearly vital, but occasionally inaccessible or even misleading.

Table 5.17 summarises the key CT differences.

iv. Diffuse cerebral abnormalities

Congenital abnormalities
(Table 5.18)

Most severe focal congenital abnormalities are readily perceived and can be analysed in terms of their location and morphology. Review of the relative proportions of the

Table 5.18
Congenital malformations of brain

1. **Neural tube closure disorders**
   Encephalocele, meningocele
2. **Disorders of neuronal migration**
   - Gyri and sulci abnormally developed in size, number or arrangement e.g. lissencephaly, polymicrogyria
   - Heterotopic grey matter
3. **Other disorders of organogenesis**
   - Agenesis of corpus callosum
   - Abnormal development of ventricles (holoprosencephaly) and related structures
   - Dandy–Walker malformation
   - Septo-optic dysplasia
4. **Chiari malformations**
5. **Phakomatoses**
   - Neurofibromatosis
   - Tuberous sclerosis
   - Sturge–Weber syndrome

supratentorial and infratentorial compartments, and assessment of midline structures for corroborative developmental lesions, may also help. More diffuse disorders such as those of neuronal migration, including lissencephaly, produce a widespread abnormality in cortical development and may be less readily appreciated. This is compounded by the relative lack of normal tissue contrast

in the incompletely myelinated paediatric brain. Poor opercularization with shallow Sylvian fissures and a consequent figure of eight appearance to the brain are useful signs. Such disorders, however, are usually accompanied by serious clinical sequelae and are referred for specialist evaluation.

Acquired

Grey–white differentiation
Generalized and focal causes of increased and decreased grey–white differentiation have been dealt with in Chapters 4 and 5. Early stages of abnormality of this type are subtle. There may be no focal disturbance of the intracerebral dynamics in the early stages, and the scan may be passed as normal.

v. The extracerebal spaces
(Fig. 5.66)

Pathology in the extracerebral spaces is most commonly related to the presence of blood or its breakdown products, or to inflammatory or neoplastic processes within the spaces.

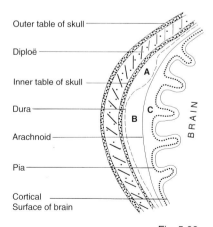

Outer table of skull
Diploë
Inner table of skull
Dura
Arachnoid
Pia
Cortical Surface of brain
BRAIN

A = Extradural collection
B = Subdural collection
C = Subarachnoid space

Fig. 5.66
Anatomical location of extracerebral collections.

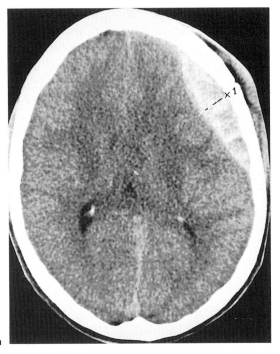

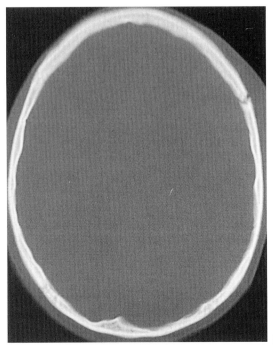

a

b

Fig. 5.67 a & b
(a) Acute extradural haematoma with (b) associated skull fracture. The collection measured 1.74 cm.

Blood and the blood products

Extradural space (Fig. 5.67)

The dura is tightly bound to the inner table of the skull, acting as a functional periosteum. A collection of blood in this potential space therefore usually requires major trauma and a high pressure local haemorrhage to strip the dura away from the skull. This accounts for the frequent association between extradural haematoma and fractures of the temporal bone crossing the middle meningeal artery. Crossing of the falx or tentorium also by definition implies an extradural location.

The collection is usually seen in the acute phase as fresh blood hyperdense to brain. It is biconvex in shape and localized to an area adjacent to the site of significant trauma. Wider windowing of this region may reveal a fracture.

Because of the risk of clot retraction and catastrophic rebleeding following the classic clinical lucid interval, these collections must be regarded with concern and referred immediately for neurosurgical assessment. They are less commonly encountered than subdural collections and recognition on the basis of their shape, characteristics and location is vital.

Subdural space

This is a true space in free communication around the neuraxis, and it frequently contains abnormal blood collections after trauma. The trauma is often less significant than that required to produce an extradural haematoma. Fractures are infrequently seen, and the bleeding may be venous and at lower pressure.

Arterial bleeding may however also produce a subdural collection, and in severe trauma a mixed pattern of blood in various spaces may be seen.

The notable physical characteristic of a subdural haematoma is its extent. It spreads through the subdural space, usually parallel with the skull vault in a crescent shape. It may be reflected over the surface of the falx or tentorium, but essentially it behaves as a layer. A thin layer under 1 cm may be reasonably tolerated by the patient, but when the haematoma exceeds 1 cm it is usually drained surgically because of the mass effect it produces on the underlying brain and which is exacerbated by any parenchymal injury to the brain. This mass effect is characteristically along a broad front, with the brain surface and cortical vessels buckled away from the vault.

The shape of the subdural collection is influenced by the turgor of the underlying brain. An atrophic brain which has lost turgor will offer little resistance to the accumulation of a collection adjacent to it, and may allow it to assume a lens rather than a crescent shape. It is for this reason that the assessment of the clinical context and the extent of the lesion are necessary in order to distinguish subdural from extradural collections.

Subdural haematomas may present promptly, but commonly the presentation is more insidious. An episode of trauma may appear to have left no obvious clinical damage, but a small collection may be present.

As the fresh blood breaks down over ensuing weeks and months, the collection may increase slightly as a result of osmotic pull. The bridging veins and small arteries spanning the normally narrow subdural space are now stretched, and vulnerable to further bleeding with decreasingly significant trauma. For this reason, subdural haematomas are often seen in the subacute, chronic and acute-on-chronic situations which may be understood by their physical characteristics.

In the acute situation, fresh blood is homogeneous and hyperdense to brain. If a clot forms, the density may increase marginally for a while, but normally the breakdown of blood products causes a progressive drop in Hu until the collection resembles water and reads in the CSF range (Fig. 5.68). Clearly there will be a time in the evolution of the collection when, as its Hu drops, it will read in a range very close to brain. The theoretical risk then exists that such an isodense collection may be missed. In practice, however, with a technically good scan, this is not an issue, as the surface of the brain has been buckled medially away from the vault in a recognizable fashion. If doubt remains, intravenous contrast can raise the Hu of the brain slightly and improve the tissue contrast, or opacify the displaced cortical veins. A developing membrane with a granulomatous reaction and neovascularity may also enhance.

Acute-on-chronic bleeds produce a heterogeneous appearance. Fluid–fluid levels may be apparent, with the fresher heavier blood products sinking with gravity. Loculations may form with membranes of varying thickness, and in the long term, dystrophic calcification may develop (Fig. 5.69).

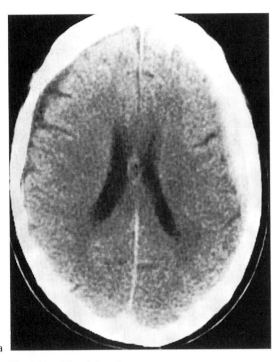

a

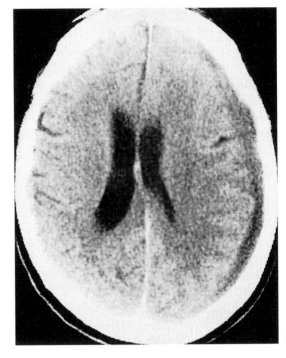

b

Fig. 5.68 a & b   (*above*)
(a) Acute shallow hyperdense subdural haematoma.
The brain surface is shifted away from the calvarium on a
broad front.
(b) Same patient 15 days later. The collection has
broken down and is now hypodense to brain, and slightly
bigger. Minimal mass effect is present on the L lateral
ventricle.

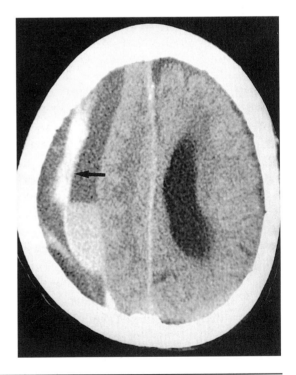

Fig. 5.69   (*right*)
Acute-on-chronic R subdural haematomas. The
collections are separated by membranes and show blood
and blood products of differing ages. The most recent
bleed shows the highest density (arrow).

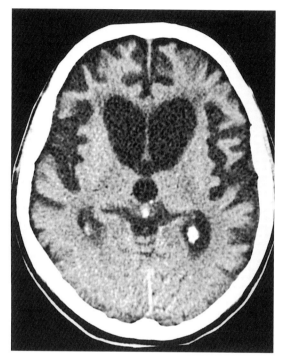

Fig. 5.70
Young demented patient with central and peripheral atrophy. The emphasis is frontal but is exaggerated by the supine position.

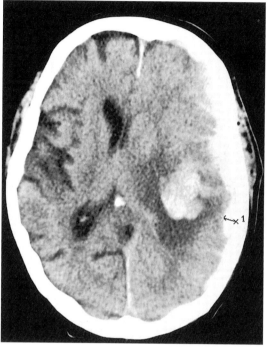

Fig. 5.71
Intraparenchymal, subdural and subarachnoid blood (within sulci) in anticoagulated patient after trauma.

Atrophy versus subdural hygroma

This issue exercises readers from time to time. When does a large amount of CSF density material over the surface of the brain represent atrophy, and when does it represent a chronic subdural collection which may need drainage? Examination of the gyri may clarify the situation. The gyral tips in atrophy are usually still in reasonable apposition to the calvarium (Fig. 5.70), whereas they will be displaced by any significant fluid collection. The appearance of the sulci will also help distinguish between atrophy and a collection. If the fluid communicates freely with gaping sulci, one is dealing with atrophy and an enlarged subarachnoid space. If the sulci

are not gaping but are being displaced across a front, the collection is subdural (Fig. 5.10). Changing the position of the head in the gantry and bringing gravity into play will also clarify the issue. The frontal sulci frequently appear more prominent than the occipital sulci in supine patients.

Subarachnoid space

Blood which enters the subarachnoid space as the result of haemorrhage from a ruptured berry aneurysm or from trauma (Fig. 5.71) will move freely throughout the subarachnoid space with the dynamic CSF circulation. Unless a block exists, blood will be identifiable in sulci, cisterns and ventricles.

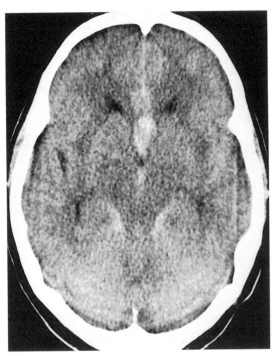

Fig. 5.72
Subarachnoid blood showing as hyperdensity within quadrigeminal, interpeduncular and ambient cisterns. A larger concentration in the anterior interhemispheric fissure suggests a ruptured anterior communicating artery aneurysm. This was confirmed angiographically.

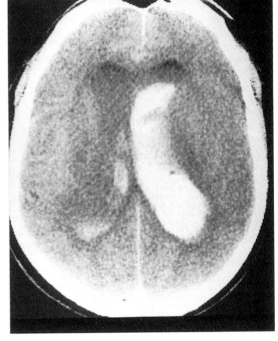

Fig. 5.73
Dense clotted blood in L lateral ventricle; blood mixed with CSF in the R lateral ventricle makes it almost isodense with brain. Clear supernatant CSF is seen anteriorly. The brain is swollen and featureless.

The heart-shaped brain stem will stand out, bathed in hyperdense blood rather than the usual CSF (Fig. 5.72). Fluid–fluid levels may be seen, with the occipital horns of the lateral ventricles being a rewarding place to search for the presence of small amounts of blood. The Sylvian fissures, the sulci and even the ventricles may 'disappear' as blood mingled with CSF raises the Hu of the fluid into the range of normal brain (Fig. 5.73).

The detection of small quantities of blood in subarachnoid haemorrhage (SAH) is a vital diagnosis. The patients are often relatively young, and may have no symptoms other than headache. A small amount of blood may be the herald bleed for a cata-strophic haemorrhage with high morbidity and mortality, and so the search should be meticulous. An exception is the rare localized perimesencephalic haemorrhage, which probably is of venous origin and has a good prognosis. The presence of mild brain swelling or hydrocephalus disturbing normal ventriculo-sulcal proportions are other useful signs in acute arterial SAH. Occasionally the source of the bleeding may be identified, in the form of an aneurysm, but angiography is still performed for definitive evaluation of the intracerebral vessels and to assess the number and condition of the aneurysms present.

If the event is more than 3 or 4 days past, blood is unlikely to be detected in the sub-

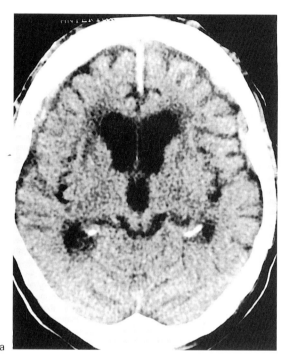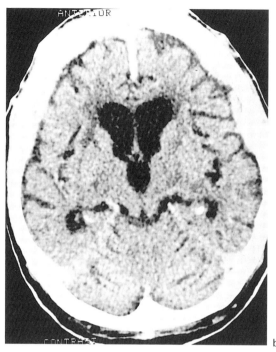

a   b

Fig. 5.74 a & b
Pre (a) and post contrast (b) scans of patient with enhancing scalp nodules and thick meningeal infiltration from secondary breast carcinoma.

arachnoid space on a head scan, and recourse must be made to lumbar puncture for the detection of xanthochromia.

Meningitis/arachnoiditis

The meninges thicken and enhance in a diffuse or nodular fashion in response to inflammation or tumour infiltration (Table 5.19). Both entities may pose difficulties for CT for two reasons.

a. Spatial resolution limits the detection of mild thickening or small nodules. Solid tumour metastases (Fig. 5.74) are more likely to be detectable than those due to lymphoma or leukaemia which are generally finer.

Table 5.19
Meningeal enhancement

> **Infections/inflammatory**
>   Bacterial, fungal, viral or parasitic meningitis
>   Neurosarcoidosis
> **Vascular**
>   Dural sinus thrombosis
> **Neoplastic**
>   Disseminated carcinoma or lymphoma

b. Contrast resolution poses difficulties as well. Small nodules may have their conspicuity increased by enhancement with intravenous agents, but inevitably are profiled against white bone where they are difficult to see. MRI, with its low signal from cortical bone, thus has a specific advantage in this regard.

If the lesions are sufficiently large, or have particularly good local contrast resolution (tumour against CSF, calcified lesions etc.), their detection will be facilitated. Commonly though, the scan is unremarkable, with lesser degrees of encroachment on normal CSF spaces not appreciated without serial imaging. The abrupt loss of normal CSF spaces such as sulci or cisterns in the presence of increasing cranial nerve signs or the reappearance of such spaces after therapy are often taken as indirect evidence of meningeal infiltration.

vi. Midline and symmetrical lesions

The search pattern for heads relies heavily on displacement of midline structures to one or other side as a consequence of focal pathology which may be space–occupying or space-creating in nature. This means that midline or symmetrical lesions are likely to be missed. This should become a conscious review area.

Midline lesions (Table 5.20)

A search of the midline structures should be part of the assessment of any head scan, to exclude the conditions listed in Table 5.20 (see also Figs. 5.75, 5.76, and 5.77).

An approach to sellar and parasellar abnormalities is given in Table 5.21.

Table 5.20
Midline lesions

Congenital lesions with midline emphasis
Disorders of diverticulation e.g. holoprosencephaly
Disorders of closure including lipoma and agenesis of corpus callosum, Chiari malformation
Other
Vein of Galen malformation
Neoplastic
Primary
Sellar/suprasellar lesions
Colloid cyst
Pineal region tumours
Medulloblastoma
Third or fourth ventricular tumours
Secondary
Pituitary stalk infiltration
Vascular
Sagittal sinus/torcular thrombosis

Symmetrical lesions

Intra-axial tumours which encase the ventricles may 'freeze' them into position and not encourage midline shift. The earliest indication may be only slight stiffening or separation of the frontal horns by mildly hyperdense material. With lesions showing little mass effect, such as optic chiasmal and optic radiation gliomatous change in neurofibromatosis, even extensive lesions may be difficult to detect on plain scans.

Multiple bilateral intra-axial lesions may set up opposing forces which counterbalance and neutralize shift (Fig. 5.78).

Extra-axial lesions which are symmetrical include neoplasms such as bilateral acoustic

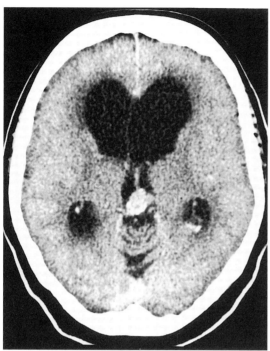

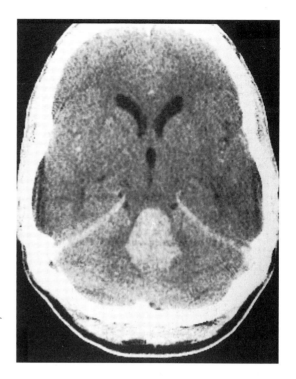

Fig. 5.75 (*above left*)
**Enhanced scan showing calcified enhanced pineal
region tumour with obstructive hydrocephalus.** Such
masses may be of pineal, germ cell or other cell origin
and can seldom be distinguished on CT characteristics
alone.

Fig. 5.76 (*above right*)
Enhancing medulloblastoma filling fourth ventricle.

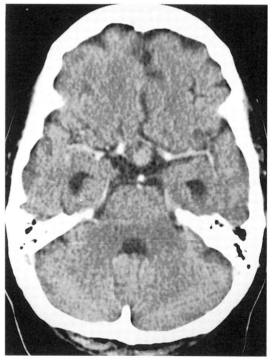

Fig. 5.77 (*right*)
**Enhanced scan showing enlarged pituitary stalk
infiltrated by metastatic breast carcinoma.**

Table 5.21
Sellar and parasellar masses

Lesion	Comment
Pituitary adenoma	
Microadenoma	– < 10 mm in diameter therefore seen best on dedicated coronal scans. Usually hypodense lesion in enhanced gland.
Macroadenoma	– > 10 mm in diameter. Fills fossa before extending into suprasellar region. Usually diffusely enhancing.
Craniopharyngioma	– Usually suprasellar. – Variable composition may commonly include calcification and/or fatty density fluid. – Bimodal incidence peaking between 5 and 10 years and in 6th decade.
Giant aneurysm of ICA	– Curvilinear rim calcification. – Marked enhancement of patent lumen.
Meningioma	– Especially middle aged women. – Hyperdense with marked contrast enhancement.
Optic chiasm glioma	– Usually in childhood. – Very rare except in patients with neurofibromatosis. – Look for involvement of optic nerve and tracts.
Metastases	– Usually in setting of known disseminated carcinoma.
Histiocytosis X	– Infiltration of pituitary infundibulum. – Usually in childhood in setting of systemic involvement. – Classic triad of diabetes insipidus, exophthalmos and lytic bone lesions (Hand–Schüller–Christian).
Hamartoma of tuber cinereum	– Nodule of neural tissue similar to normal hypothalamus usually attached to tuber cinereum or mammillary bodies by a pedicle. – No enhancement. – Usually an incidental finding. – Do not grow on follow up.

Germ cell tumours/teratomas	– Usually childhood and young adults.
	– Germinoma.
	  – least differentiated.
	  – usually homogeneous and enhance.
	  – may be metastatic from primary in pineal region.
	– Teratoma – look for fat and ossified components.

Dermoid/epidermoid	– Dermoid
	  – Childhood.
	  – Heterogeneous and commonly contain fat or fat–fluid levels.
	– Epidermoid
	  – 4th and 5th decades.
	  – Usually laterally in basal cisterns and especially CP angle.
	  – Density only slightly different to CSF. No enhancement.

Table 5.21
Cont'd

Lesion	Comment
Empty sella	– Common normal finding. – Fossa filled with CSF density. – Look for pituitary infundibulum extending down to floor of fossa.
Cranial nerve neuroma	– Epicentre lateral to sella and commonly from Meckel's cave. – Diffuse contrast enhancement.
Chordoma	– Usually arises inferior to sella with prominent bony involvement of clivus. – Variably calcified.

schwannomas in central neurofibromatosis. Here the brain stem and the fourth ventricle may be compressed and deformed from both sides. There are usually other stigmata of the disease. Bilateral extracerebral collections such as chronic subdural haematomas are a more practical problem, but the displaced cortical surfaces hold the answer in this condition. With such lesions, the lateral ventricles are also compressed towards the midline and have the natural curves of their frontal and occipital horns reduced ('parenthesis' ventricles).

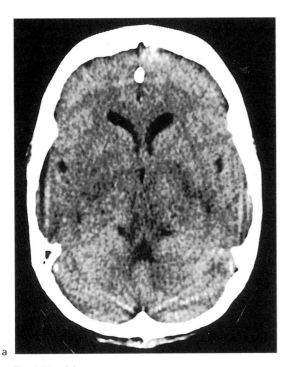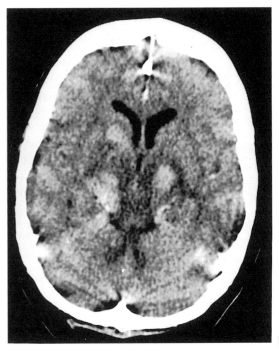

a

b

Fig. 5.78 a & b
(a) Plain and (b) enhanced scan of patient with multiple intra-axial deposits of NHL, which can be protean in its manifestations. The clues are the ventriculo-sulcal disproportionality, and the compression deformity of V3.

Bibliography

Atlas S W 1990 Adult supratentorial tumours. Seminars in Roentgenology XXV(2): 130–154

Barkovich A J, Kjos B O, Norman D, Edwards M S 1989 Revised classification of posterior fossa cysts and cystlike malformations based on the results of multiplanar MRI imaging. American Journal of Neuroradiology 10: 977–988

Bilaniuk L T 1990 Adult infratentorial tumours. Seminars in Roentgenology XXV(2): 155–173

Bird C R, Drayer B P, Gilles F 1989 Pathophysiology of 'reverse' edema in global cerebral ischaemia. American Journal of Neuroradiology 10: 95–98

Boyko D B, Cooper D F, Grossman C B 1991 Contrast-enhanced CT of isodense subdural hematoma. American Journal of Neuroradiology 12: 341–343

Caresio J F, McMillan J H, Balnitzsky S 1991 Coexistent intra- and extracranial mass lesions: an unusual manifestation of histiocytosis X. American Journal of Neuroradiology 12: 82

Castillo M, Scatliff J H, Bouldin T W, Suzuki K 1992 Radiologic–pathologic correlation: intracranial astrocytoma. American Journal of Neuroradiology 13: 1609–1616

Chang T, Teng M M H, Guo W–Y, Sheng W C 1989 CT of pineal tumours and intracranial germ cell tumours. American Journal of Neuroradiology 10: 1039–1044

Cormier P J, Long E R, Russell E J 1992 MR Imaging of posterior fossa infarctions: vascular territories and clinical correlates. Radiographics 12: 1079–1096.

Davis P C, Hudgins P A, Peterman S B, Hoffman J C 1991 Diagnosis of cerebral metastases. Double-dose delayed CT vs. contrast-enhanced MR imaging. American Journal of Neuroradiology 12: 293–300

Drayer BP 1988 Imaging of the aging brain. Parts 1 and 2. Radiology 166: 785–906.

Eisenberg R L 1994 Skull and spine imaging. Raven Press, New York

Fitz C R 1982 Midline anomalies of the brain and spine. Radiologic Clinics of North America 20(1): 95–104

George A E 1991 Chronic communicating hydrocephalus and periventricular white matter disease: a debate with regard to cause and effect. American Journal of Neuroradiology 12: 42–44

Ho V B, Smirniotopoulous J G, Murphy F M, Rushing E J 1992 Radiologic–pathologic correlation: hemangioblastoma. American Journal of Neuroradiology 13: 1343–1352

Hoe J 1989 CT of nasopharyngeal carcinoma: significance of widening of preoccipital soft tissue on axial scans. American Journal of Roentgenology 153: 867–872

Imaging in Ophthalmology Part I. Editor Mafee M F 1987 Radiologic Clinics of North America

Imaging in Ophthalmology Part II. Editor Mafee M F 1987 Radiologic Clinics of North America

Jelinek J, Smirniotopoulous J G, Parisi J E, Kanzer M 1990 Lateral ventricular neoplasms of the brain: differential diagnosis based on clinical, CT and MR findings. American Journal of Neuroradiology 11: 567–574

Jinkins J R 1991 Clinical manifestations of hydrocephalus caused by impingement of the corpus callosum on the falx: an MR study in 40 patients. American Journal of Neuroradiology 12: 331–340

Kaplan S B, Kemp S S, Oh K S 1991 Radiographic manifestations of bony anomalies of the skull. Radiologic Clinics of North America 29(2): 195–218

Kirkwood JR 1990 Essentials of Neuroimaging. Churchill Livingstone, New York

Kollias S S, Ball W S, Prenger E C 1993 Cystic malformations of the posterior fossa: differential diagnosis clarified through embryologic analysis. Radiographics 13(6): 1211–31

Lee Y-Y, Tien R D, Bruner J M, DePena C A, van Tassel P 1989 Loculated intracranial leptomeningeal metastases: CT & MR characteristics. American Journal of Neuroradiology 10: 1171–1179

Lee Y-Y, Van Tassel P 1989 Intracranial oligodendrogliomas: imaging findings in 35 untreated cases. American Journal of Neuroradiology 10: 119–127

Lee Y-Y, van Tassel P, Bruner J M, Moser R P, Shane J C 1989 Juvenile pilocytic astrocytomas: CT and MR characteristics. American Journal of Neuroradiology 10: 363–370

Maeder P P, Holtas S L, Basibüyük L N et al 1990 Colloid cysts of the 3rd ventricle: correlation of MR and CT findings with histology and chemical analysis. American Journal of Roentgenology 155: 135–141

Mirvis S E, Wolf A L, Namagucki Y, Corradino G, Joslyn

J N 1990 Post-traumatic cerebral infarction diagnosed by CT: prevalence, origin and outcome. American Journal of Neuroradiology 11: 355–360

Rinkel G J E, Wijdicks E F M, Vermeulen M et al 1991 Non aneurysmal perimesencephalic subarachnoid hemorrhage: CT and MR patterns that differ from aneurysmal rupture. American Journal of Neuroradiology 12: 829–839

Román G C 1991 White matter lesions and normal pressure hydrocephalus: Binswanger disease or Hakim syndrome. American Journal of Neuroradiology 12: 40–41

Sage M R 1982 Blood–brain barrier: phenomenon of increasing importance to the imaging clinician. American Journal of Neuroradiology 3: 127–138

Sarwar M 1989 The septum pellucidum: normal and abnormal. American Journal of Neuroradiology 10: 989–1005

Sato Y, Kao S C S, Smith W L 1991 Radiographic manifestations of anomalies of the brain. Radiologic Clinics of North America 29(2): 179–194

Sheporaitis L A, Osborn A G, Smirniotopoulos J G, Clunie D A, Howieson J, D'Agostino A N 1992 Intracranial meningioma. American Journal of Neuroradiology 13: 29–37

Smirniotopoulous J G, Murphy F M 1992 The phakomatoses. American Journal of Neuroradiology 13: 725–746

Smith R R 1990 Brain stem tumours. Seminars in Roentgenology XXV(31): 249–262

Spoto G R, Press G A, Hesselink J R, Solomon R 1990 Intracranial ependymoma and subependymoma: MR manifestations. American Journal of Roentgenology 154: 837–845

Tomsick T A, Brott T G, Chambers A A et al 1990 Hyperdense middle cerebral artery sign on CT: efficacy in detecting MCA thrombosis. American Journal of Neuroradiology 11: 473–477

Truwit C L, Barkovich A J 1990 Pathogenesis of intracranial lipoma: an MR study in 42 patients. American Journal of Roentgenology 155: 855–864

Valk P E, Dillon W P 1991 Radiation injury of the brain. American Journal of Neuroradiology 12: 45–62

Van Tassel P, Lee Y, Bruner J M 1986 Supratentorial ependymomas: computed tomographic and pathologic correlations. Journal of Computed Tomography 10: 157–165

Yock D H 1991 Imaging of CNS disease, 2nd edn. Mosby-Year Book, St Louis

Yoshino M T, Lucro R 1992 Pleomorphic xanthoastrocytoma. American Journal of Neuroradiology 13: 1330–1332

Zimmerman R A 1990 Imaging of intrasellar, suprasellar and parasellar tumours. Seminars in Roentgenology XXV(2): 174–197

Zülch K-J 1985 The cerebral infarct. Springer, Berlin

CHAPTER 6

Extending the search pattern

Once the intracranial contents have been examined, the search pattern should be extended to any of the following areas which may have been included in the scan either by chance or design. Inflammatory and malignant pathology has many routes by which pathologic processes may spread from one region to another. These include spread through natural foramina and vascular connections particularly in the skull base and pterygopalatine fossae, and also direct invasion through bone.

Skull base

It is our practice even in routine examinations of the head to scan the skull base with finer slices (5 mm rather than 10 mm) and to photograph these on bone and soft tissue windows. Widening the window will improve discrimination of cortical and medullary bony detail and deal with the wider range of tissue densities which need to be distinguished in this region.

Special review areas include the cribriform plate, the clivus for lesions such as chordoma; the foramen lacerum and related basal skull neural exit foramina (Table 3.1) which are eroded amongst others by nasopharyngeal carcinomas anteriorly, and posteriorly by glomus jugulare tumours (Fig. 6.1), and the foramen magnum in the midline for congenital assimilation anomalies such as occipitalization of upper cervical vertebrae.

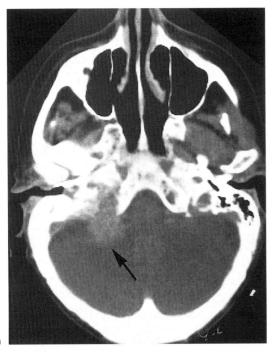

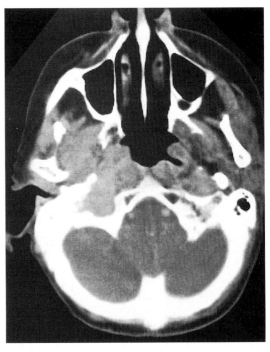

a

b

Fig. 6.1 a & b
Enhanced scans showing a glomus jugulare tumour which had its epicentre in the jugular fossa. (a) There is extensive aggressive bony destruction and an intracranial component (arrow), as well as anterior spread through the skull base to the nasopharynx. (b) The normal paired recesses and fatty parapharyngeal space seen on the L have been obliterated on the R.

The sella and juxtasellar regions are common sites for masses (Table 5.21). More detailed scanning and special windowing is needed to assess bone destruction and calcification in patterns which will aid differential diagnosis. The preservation of the ghost of a sella suggests a mass of pituitary origin. Smooth, well marginated bone erosion is a sign of an indolent process (Fig. 6.2) whereas aggressive lesions such as chordomas will produce a more ragged pattern. Residual fragments of bone may be difficult to distinguish from a destructive calcifying mass. The cavernous sinus and its dural reflections must be assessed. Local dural thickening or stalk infiltration are further useful discriminating features.

Orbits

The scan planes generally used these days run parallel to the floor of the anterior cranial fossa. This allows improved visualization of posterior fossa structures and also spares the lens from radiation. In most cases, therefore, the orbit will be imaged incompletely if at all.

Occasionally, though, a more truly axial orientation or more inferior slices will be used and the orbit will be included in the head examination.

The orbital contents should be symmetrical. An old exenteration with prosthetic replacement may not have been mentioned in the history. The location of the globes in relation to the facial skeleton should be

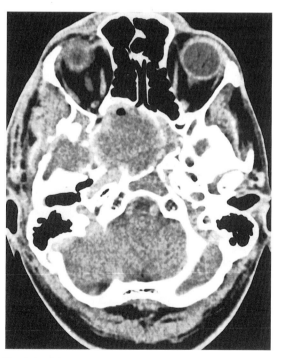
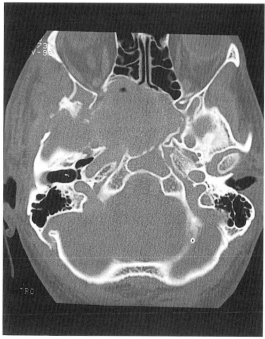

a

b

Fig. 6.2 a & b
Chronic pituitary abscess. (a) Enhancing cystic mass with small gas collection anteriorly. (b) Extensive bone thinning and destruction in a pattern of indolent expansion.

assessed for proptosis or enophthalmos, but minor degrees will be more obvious to the patient than the radiologist. The lenses should be normally located.

Any mass lesion or space-occupying process should be analysed in terms of its anatomic location: within the globe or the retrobulbar tissues; within the muscle cone or extra-conal in location (Table 6.1). The precise relationship to the lacrimal gland, the optic nerve and other readily identifiable structures should be sought.

Specific anatomic location is so important that it is worthy of further effort, such as coronal slices if the issue cannot be resolved

Table 6.1
Orbital pathology

Arising within the orbit
- Intraocular e.g. retinoblastoma, melanoma, metastases (lung and breast)
- Intraconal
    - Vascular lesions e.g. haemangioma, lymphangioma, varices
    - Tumours
        Related to optic nerve e.g. glioma, meningioma
        Other as for intraocular lesions above
    - Inflammatory/infiltrative
        Pseudotumour, amyloid,
            Erdheim–Chester disease
    - Traumatic
        Foreign body, haematoma
- Extraconal or muscular
    - Inflammatory as above but also thyroid myopathy, orbital myositis, dacryocystitis
    - Neoplastic
        Benign tumours associated with any of the orbital contents including muscles, nerves, lacrimal glands etc.
        Lymphoma, Burkitt's tumour.
Arising extraorbitally
- From nose, nasopharynx, paranasal sinus, orbital bone and infratemporal fossa, e.g. fibrous dysplasia, bony neoplasms, soft tissue tumours (carcinomas), granulomatous disease.
- From intracranial pathology e.g. encephalomeningocele, carotid-cavernous fistula, tumour extension especially meningioma

on axial images alone. One classic trap involves the sandwich formed by superior and inferior rectus muscles with the optic nerve between them. Although these structures converge at the orbital apex they follow a more parallel course in the mid and anterior orbit and can be mistaken for each other (Fig. 6.3). An expanded muscle belly is likely to be due to an infiltrative condition such as a thyroid myopathy, while an expanded optic nerve may represent a tumour such as glioma or meningioma. The optic nerve has some redundancy to allow for upward and downward gaze, and may therefore be sectioned incompletely in axial images giving a false impression of its true dimensions. Again, scans at right angles in the coronal plane will resolve the issue.

The natural tissue contrast of the orbit is exceptionally good. The structures cover a wide range of Hu, from the water of the vitreous humour to the soft tissue of the muscles and nerves and the abundant retrobulbar fat, with everything encased in the bony skeleton of the orbit. Tissue discrimination is therefore good as well as easy. Intravenous contrast adds little in routine cases, but may help to clarify the nature of an observed abnormality. Dynamic manoeuvres such as a Valsalva may engorge a vascular malformation or varix.

Any lesion approaching the orbital apex should prompt careful assessment of intracranial extension via the optic canal or orbital fissures. Meningiomas, optic gliomas and retinoblastomas are all capable of doing this, and intravenous contrast is useful in enhancing these intracranial extensions against brain.

Even if the patient has an orbital presentation, the source of the problem may be in the paranasal sinuses or infratemporal fossa.

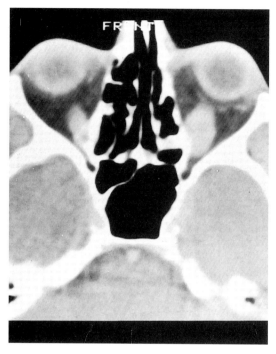

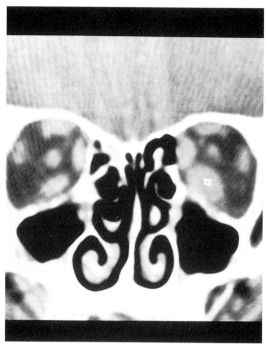

a

b

Fig. 6.3 a & b
Axial scan (a) shows a fusiform intra-orbital mass which could be interpreted as an optic nerve glioma. Coronal scan (b) shows it to be asymmetric infiltration of the inferior rectus muscle. The patient had thyroid myopathy.

Mass lesions arising in the orbit, or from the adjacent structures such as the paranasal sinuses, will generally produce proptosis in proportion to their bulk. An important exception is metastatic breast carcinoma, which may be so desmoplastic as to present with the unusual combination of abnormal soft tissue and enopthalmos.

Paranasal sinuses

Mass lesions originating in the paranasal sinuses may erode through relatively thin areas of the orbital bony skeleton, such as the medial wall (lamina papyracea) or the orbital roof, to cause proptosis. Conditions causing this include inflammatory processes of acute or chronic nature, and neoplasms.

Mucoceles deserve a special mention, due to their indolent nature and smooth erosion of bone. If more than 1 sinus is involved, the mucoceles may show opacity of different attenuation values, reflecting differing viscosity of their contents (Fig. 6.4).

Commonly, CT in sinus disease shows only a non-specific opacity in the sinus in question, and the differentiation between tenacious high density secretions in an inflammatory process and soft tissue lesions such as neoplasms is not possible. Where the two coexist, as in a paranasal sinus carcinoma which occludes a draining ostium and produces an obstructive mucocele, this inability to distinguish tumour margin from mucus on CT is frustrating. Recourse must usually be made to MRI for precise ana-

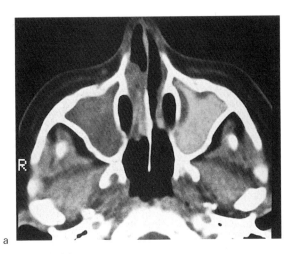
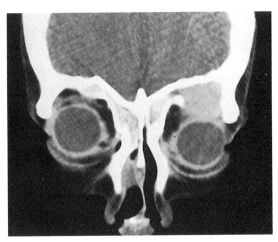

a

b

Fig. 6.4 a & b
**Plain axial (a) and coronal (b) of patient with multiple paranasal sinus mucoceles, with pus of differing
viscosities and consequently differing Hu.** The most inspissated collection (L antral) reads in the soft tissue range.
The L frontal lesion has eroded the orbital roof and displaced the globe.

tomic staging. The closer the Hu of the tumour and the mucus are, the more difficult the distinction will be on CT. If a significant difference does exist it will be best seen on narrow window settings.

A wide setting (around 2000 Hu) is optimal for studying details of bone and particularly the patterns of bone destruction.

Spread of sinus and particularly antral pathology through the postero-lateral wall into the retroantral fat pad, or up into the pterygomaxillary fissure, should also be sought, as this too has sinister implications and correlates more strongly with tumour.

Nasopharynx

As with paranasal sinuses, primary nasopharyngeal pathology may first be detected on a head scan as a result of transcranial spread.

The search pattern for this area must include identification of the normal paired recesses of the nasopharynx, and the important parapharyngeal fat plane which runs obliquely through the nasopharynx and demarcates the muscles of mastication from those of deglutition. Any blurring or displacement of the normal fat planes, either here or in the prevertebral space, must be explained.

The fossa of Rosenmüller is the epicentre for nasopharyngeal carcinoma with its penchant for submucosal and perineural spread. The anterior recess marks the exit of the Eustachian tube and should be checked in patients presenting with unusual or intractable middle ear disease (Fig. 6.5). The nasopharynx is rich in lymphoid tissue (Waldeyer's ring) and may show symmetric encroachment by enlarged adenoids or lymphomatous nodes. Such encroachment may appear very orderly and be underestimated. As a rule of thumb, the lateral boundaries of the normal nasopharynx should parallel the medial pterygoid plates.

Midline lesions in the nasopharynx are most commonly cystic notochordal remnants (Thornwald cysts), but more sinister

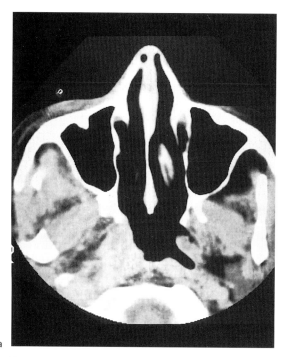 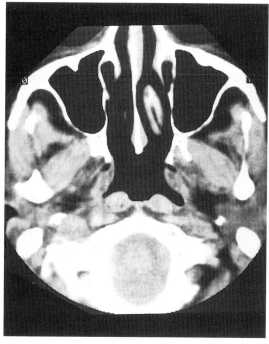

a   b

Fig. 6.5 a & b
Patient with recurrent recent middle ear disease and blood dyscrasia. Initial scan (a) shows soft tissue mass obliterating the normal recess for the Eustachian tube and the more posterior fossa of Rosenmüller on the R. There is also infiltration of the R retroantral fat. Biopsy showed leukaemic cells. Three weeks later (b) the deposits have melted with treatment.

processes involving the clivus or skull base and extending as mass lesions into the nasopharynx must be excluded. These include chordomas, chondrosarcomas, plasmacytomas and other skull base neoplasms.

The ear and petrous region (Fig. 3.4)

External ear

Opacities within the external canal usually represent wax and, more rarely, destructive conditions such as otitis externa.

Middle ear

Depending on the fineness of the slices used, the middle and inner ear are variably displayed. Symmetry of bony development is important, to exclude congenital anomalies of the bony canals of the great vessels such as the carotid. When the bony walls are defective, a pulsatile tinnitus may be produced and mimic the presentation of a glomus tympanicum tumour, with potentially disastrous results.

The drums should be symmetrical; not thickened, bowed or retracted. The middle ear cavity should contain air, and a symmetrical group of ossicles should be identified. While the anatomy is complex, it is comforting that the range of common acquired pathology is limited. The commonest type is middle ear infection, which may progress to secondary cholesteatoma formation. The lateral attic spur (scutum) and ossicles are eroded, and cavities form in the mastoid, lined or filled with abnormal soft tissue.

Inner ear

Visible detail again depends on the fineness of slices used and the photographic display utilized. A detailed description of congenital or acquired pathology is beyond the scope of this book, but comparison should be made of left and right sides for gross symmetry of development, degree of mineralization, and any foci of destruction.

A particular note of caution should be sounded regarding the internal auditory canal. The normal situation is to have the bony canal visualized with parallel, well-defined walls. Minor degrees of flaring or trumpeting of the medial end are, however, very common, and in the vast majority of cases not due to the presence of an acoustic Schwannoma. Another way of looking at this is to remember that fewer than 5% of patients with unilateral hearing loss have acoustic Schwannomas, and of those who do, three quarters have associated disequilibrium or tinnitus. This should help to triage those patients who need referral for MRI. If such a tumour is indeed present, and is large enough to have caused pressure erosion, projection of its circumference will suggest a lesion of sufficient size to be identified readily with intravenous contrast and fine slices (2 mm or less). If the flaring is bilateral, the possibility of bilateral Schwannoma is negligible, unless the patient has Type II neurofibromatosis (NF). Dural ectasia without tumours may be seen in NF Type I.

The mastoid air cells should also form part of the normal search pattern. In the acute situation, haziness of the mastoid air cells may indicate acute infection which may precipitate a cerebral presentation by caus-

ing deep venous or venous sinus thrombosis. In cases of trauma, opacity of the air cells due to blood may be the first indication of a petrous or skull base fracture.

Coarsening and sclerosis of the mastoid air cells indicate chronic infection. Bone destruction usually indicates cholesteatoma formation as an extension through the aditus of chronic middle ear disease. In this context, the postoperative ear poses a unique problem in the assessment of recurrent disease. The surgical cavity should be smoothly marginated and clean. The presence of ragged soft tissue usually implies recurrent cholesteatoma. The coronal projection aids in the appreciation of anatomy and also in the assessment of possible fistulation to the semi-circular canals or destruction of the axially-oriented bony tegmen tympani.

Cranial vault and coverings

The best assessment of the cranial vault is made on the scout film, as noted in Chapter 3.

The scalp may show skin thickening, bruising or laceration in cases of injury; benign nodules such as sebaceous cysts or neurofibromas, or malignant tumour deposits.

Rarely, opaque foreign material in the hair may produce unusual artefacts on axial images.

Vertebrae and craniocervical junction

The upper cervical vertebrae are usually visible on the scout film and must be checked in cases of trauma (Fig. 4.2). Assimilation anomalies may also be visible, and occasionally mass lesions at the cranio-cervical junction. At the cervico-medullary junction, at the level of the foramen magnum, a generous pool of low-density CSF usually surrounds the cord, allowing it and the lower limits of the cerebellar tonsils to be distinguished.

Face

Major injuries, tumours or rampant infections of the face and its skeleton are frequently accompanied by intracranial pathology. If slices through the head are to be continued inferiorly into the face, the anatomy will be easier to recognize if a true axial rather than an angled orientation is used. Because of the multiple thin plates of bone which run in the axial plane to form the facial skeleton, coronal imaging is of particular value in determining anatomic relationships and assessing fractures and displacement.

Facial fat, aerated sinuses and bone in combination produce, as in the orbit, excellent natural tissue contrast.

CHAPTER 7

Pitfalls and normal variants in cranial CT

Inherent in the technique of scanning

Partial volume
Partial volume averaging may cause a structure to be partially averaged 'into' or 'out of' a slice or a voxel (see Chapter 2).

Streak artefact/beam hardening
This includes the characteristic interpetrous artefact (Chapter 2), and other streak artefacts seen as a result of irregularities along the inner table of the skull. These artefacts can be reduced with finer slices, using slice summation techniques, or made less obvious by widening the window.

Inappropriate slice prescription
Pathology may be missed if there are insufficient slices or if they are too thick for the detail required.

Inherent in technique of photography

The windowing may have been inappropriate to discriminate structures at either extreme of the grey scale. In the head, the most common problems follow failure to use a wide window to interrogate bone.

Artefactual

Artefacts in CT are fortunately few and generally easy to recognize. They include those due to mechanical or physiological problems or the presence of foreign material. Material such as metal is of extremely high density and produces severe streak artefacts. A more subtle pitfall is presented when the material is plastic, silastic or wood which are closer to the Hounsfield range for normal tissues and may not be recognized for what they are. The detectability of such material depends on its mass, its electron density, its inherent contrast against the tissues in which it is embedded, and the secondary effects associated with its presence such as anatomic disruption or distortion.

Real structures and normal variants

Real pathological structures such as symmetrical and midline lesions (Chapter 5) cause perceptual difficulty, as do lesions with mixed patterns of space occupation and space creation. There is however a larger group of pitfalls where the problem is analysis rather than perception. Many of these will prove to be normal structures or normal variants.

The list of normal variants grows steadily, with further observation and clinical correlations redefining the boundaries of normality.

Normal structures which have not been recognized as such have presented pitfalls as each generation becomes accustomed to the new frontiers in spatial and contrast resolution.

They are best discussed in anatomic terms, as follows.

Skull
Most of the unusual appearances of the skull may be dismissed as normal variants if the underlying brain appears normally developed.

Shape
Plagiocephaly produces an asymmetric skull where axial images may still result in paired structures not being equally displayed on any one slice. If one cranial subcompart-

ment, such as the middle cranial fossa, looks small, examination of the adjacent slices will give a more valid idea of whether it truly is reduced in size or whether it simply spans a different group of contiguous images.

Protuberances and scalloping

Frontal hyperostosis is characteristically lumpy and spares the midline. The additional bone should be well marginated and of normal texture. Focal protuberant sclerosis may also be seen along normal suture lines.

Local bony overgrowth or over-pneumatization in nearby air cells or sinuses, if pathological, will be seen with maldevelopment or hypoplasia of underlying brain. If the underlying brain is normal, the calvarial changes are most likely normal variants without significance. These include variations of sphenoid, clinoid, petrous tip and mastoid air cell development. A lack of sclerosis or of associated soft tissue opacity points to such appearances as being normal variants. Smooth scalloping of the inner table is also seen, particularly in association with large, dominant dural sinuses.

Fenestrations and areas of thinning

Large diploic channels and emissary foramina are common in the parietal and occipital regions. They are well circumscribed and smoothly marginated and may have identifiable vessels or venous sinuses associated with them.

Normal bony channels, notably the superior orbital fissures, may commonly be asymmetric without being abnormal.

Areas of thinning of the calvarium are often seen in the parietal bone and in the temporal squama, also without being of significance.

Partial volume averaging

Parts of the irregular floor of the anterior cranial fossa or the arcuate eminence of the petrous ridge may project into a slice and be mistaken for haemorrhage or calcification. The solution is to check the next slice inferiorly, or confirm the bony nature of the density by reading the Hu. Coronal imaging will help in distinguishing frontal contusions from such bony projections in cases of trauma.

The jugular tubercles and the planum sphenoidale can be resolved using the same techniques.

Flaring of the internal auditory canals (IAC)

See Chapter 6.

Intracranial
Focal calcific densities

Physiological calcifications in paired structures such as the basal ganglia and the petroclinoid ligaments usually occur symmetrically. Occasionally a calcified petroclinoid ligament may be mistaken for a calcified vessel, but its course is oblique rather than circumferential around the brainstem. Even quite extensive calcification in the extrapyramidal system may be unassociated with clinical abnormalities, though there are pathologic, usually metabolic conditions where the appearance is similar (Chapter 5). Simple biochemical blood testing is the first step if clinical doubt exists.

Heavy calcific deposits in the periventricular region have been mistaken for haemorrhage, but an ROI measurement will resolve this. The lack of acute neurologic abnormality is another pointer to calcification rather than blood.

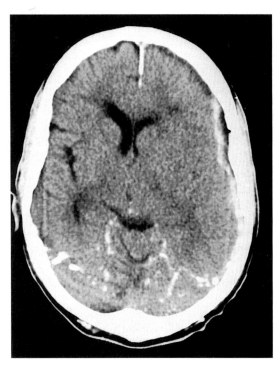

Fig. 7.1
Extensive calcification in the falx anteriorly, and over the surface of the tentorium. Its physical characteristics are different even to the naked eye from the small fresh L subdural haematoma which is producing mass effect.

Even if an ROI cannot be performed, calcification has a characteristically hard, bright and brittle appearance which can be helpful when it occurs in unusual morphology as it may do, for example, in the tentorium (Fig. 7.1).

Ventricles, cisterns and choroid

Normal ventricular asymmetry has been dealt with elsewhere.

Calcified choroid is commonly seen in the trigones, but occasionally heavy calcification is also present in the choroid plexus of the third ventricle, in the temporal horns, or extending laterally through the foramina of Luschka of the fourth ventricle. The choroid

should enhance mildly and symmetrically, with abnormal enhancement suggesting infection, tumour seeding or recent haemorrhage.

The cavum septum pellucidum is seen in neonates but may persist into adult life with its extension posterior to the foramen of Monro known as a cavum vergae (Fig. 7.2). Such cava are usually asymptomatic, but a higher incidence has been observed in boxers who have suffered repeated head trauma and who may have other symptoms of brain damage. In normal individuals these fluid-filled spaces should not be under pressure, should not obstruct adjacent ventricles, and should contain fluid of CSF density. This will distinguish them from entities such as lipomas of the corpus callosum.

The cistern of the lamina terminalis may be seen between the frontal horns, and should not be mistaken for the posterior extension of the anterior interhemispheric fissure which is allowed to develop in callosal agenesis.

The cisterna magna may be prominent, but also should be of CSF density and not in obvious communication with the fourth ventricle. Occasionally there may be some vermian hypoplasia, but more commonly the underlying brain is normal, and there should certainly be no mass or neurologic defect.

Pools of CSF may be seen just cephalad to the normal vermis in the superior cerebellar cistern.

The supracornual cleft of the temporal horn may project as a small hypodensity close to the internal capsule and be mistaken for a lacunar infarct. If doubt exists, additional fine slices will show it is not rounded in its third dimension but communicates with the ventricular system. Occasionally the posterior extent of the Sylvian fissure will

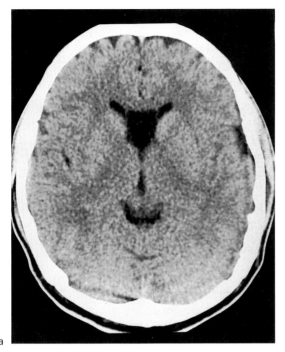
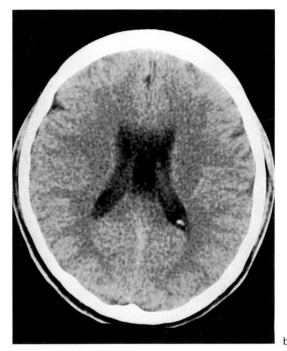

a

b

Fig. 7.2 a & b
Cavum septum pellucidum (a) and vergae (b).

also contain more CSF than its anterior extent, with similar misinterpretation as an infarct. These are however usually young patients with small CSF spaces and an inappropriate setting for infarction.

Meninges and reflections

The dura, especially in its tentorial reflection, may be thickened or calcified to the point of appearing quite substantial. The presence of large pools of dense blood in the dural sinuses, and of normal enhancement, also contribute to these being mistaken for pathology.

Vessels and perivascular spaces

The pericallosal arteries and the basilar artery frequently follow undulating courses without necessarily being displaced for pathological reasons. Inspection of surrounding structures will exclude pathology either pushing or tethering these vessels. A dominant vertebral artery, often the left, is another common variation of normal.

A large vein of Galen may be shown as a smooth oval to linear structure, depending on the angle of the scan. Contributions from the internal cerebral veins and veins of Rosenthal may be identifiable in the surrounding quadrigeminal plate cistern, but challenge with intravenous contrast will produce a typical vascular opacification pattern if any doubt remains.

Prominent Virchow–Robin or perivascular spaces have been recognized with increasing frequency on scanners with good spatial resolution. They are especially noticeable around the penetrating branches of the middle cerebral arteries and should also not be mistaken for lacunar infarcts.

Normal parenchymal structures

Normal parenchymal structures, especially those which enhance slightly with intravenous contrast, may be perceived as abnormal. Chief of these are the flocculus, occasionally mistaken for a cerebellopontine angle mass, and the vermis, mistaken for a tumour indenting the fourth ventricle. Correlation with clinical findings, more detailed slices, and no corroborative pathophysiological findings should rule these out.

The limitations of CT

The CT revolution has not yet run its course. Further technological improvements are expected which will produce clearer images and in shorter times. MRI and other in vivo neurophysiological imaging will allow us better correlation with CT, and our understanding of the structure and function of the human brain looks set to continue growing for the foreseeable future.

So why does CT not provide us with a higher proportion of the answers in clinical dilemmas even now? It may be that the visible CT manifestations are non-specific in a particular patient at a particular point in time. It may be that the lesion is beyond the limits of perception and consequently of analysis. Possible reasons for this are listed below. Most importantly, however, it is because of the difficulties in clinical correlation, and some of these are listed too, in the certain knowledge that the list will grow as our knowledge does.

Areas of perceptual limitation with CT
Small lesions

Lesions may be so small as to be below the spatial resolution capability of CT.

Isodense lesions

- Lesions closely resembling brain e.g. grade I astrocytomas, isodense subdurals, early demyelinating plaques.
- Lesions where the changes are metabolic and not yet anatomically visible e.g. early infarction. CT diagnosis still depends largely on a disturbance of structure rather than function.

Diffuse lesions

This is a perceptual problem (see Chapter 5).

Lesions in difficult anatomic locations

- Posterior fossa lesions, due to interpetrous artefact.
- High convexity lesions.

Leptomeningeal pathology (see Chapter 5)

Clinical correlation and CT

Much of clinical neurology has traditionally been based on the eliciting of a constellation of physical signs which in concert suggest a certain anatomic location for the lesion. The advent of CT has produced many surprising cases where the clinical and imaging correlation has not appeared to be firm. This should not discourage clinicians from attempting to give working diagnoses wherever possible so that the radiologist can tailor the scan appropriately.

The following include some of the reasons for difficulties in clinical correlation.

Lesion location and intracranial associations

In any particular constellation of signs, a subgroup may dominate which mislead the clinician as to the precise location or extent of the lesion. The complexities of association pathways and influences are also not yet fully understood.

These include the phenomenon of transient contralateral cerebellar signs in patients with supratentorial lesions (crossed cerebellar diaschisis) and the hypertrophic olivary degeneration which may follow cerebellar haemorrhage. New techniques of in vivo neurophysiological study will doubtless reveal many more examples.

Lesion number

Multiple lesions may produce a mixed picture which is difficult to interpret.

Nonspecificity of symptoms

Non-specific symptoms such as confusion can be produced by a variety of vastly differing pathologies, from Alzheimer's disease and encephalitis to sagittal sinus thrombosis with venous infarction. Detailed history and examination will clarify these with time, but at first presentation the information may be incomplete.

Evolution

How rapidly a lesion develops, how much oedema it excites and how quickly it resolves can all account for fluctuating and unstable clinical pictures.

False localizing signs

Cranial nerves with long extra-axial intracranial courses, such as the VIth, are vulnerable to the effects of remote lesions displacing intracerebral contents.

Contre-coup lesions

In head injuries the contre-coup phenomenon frequently produces signs in an area remote from the region of major trauma.

Extracranial influences

Over- or underhydration, intercurrent infection and medications can all influence the level of consciousness, especially in older patients, and limit precise clinical and imaging correlations.

Bibliography

Kuhns L R, Seeger J 1983 Atlas of computed tomography variants. Year Book, Chicago

Reivich M 1992 Crossed cerebellar diaschisis – commentary. American Journal of Neuroradiology 13: 62–64

Revel M P, Mann M, Brugieres P, Poirier J, Gaston A 1991 MR appearance of hypertrophic olivary degeneration after contralateral cerebellar hemorrhage. American Journal of Neuroradiology 12: 71–72

Vogler J B, Helms C A, Callen P W 1986 Normal variants and pitfalls in imaging. Saunders, Philadelphia

CHAPTER 8

Applying the principles

Case
1

Fig. 8.1 (a–d)

Clinical problem

This 57-year-old woman was found unconscious. The scout view and 3 non-enhanced representative images are shown.

Image analysis

a. The scout image provides valuable evidence by showing a craniotomy flap and a metallic clip consistent with the surgical treatment of an aneurysm in the past.

b–d. Where is the pathology and what is its nature?

There are multiple abnormalities, both intra- and extra-axial. These have caused gross distortion of the normal ventricular configuration.

The major focal lesion is a large L frontal space-occupying process with the density of fresh blood. This has caused L to R midline shift and effaced the sulci.

There are well circumscribed hypodense areas with CSF density in the R hemisphere which is the side of the craniotomy flap. Following them through the anatomic sequence confirms that they are part of a dilated R lateral ventricle. The surgery suggests there may have been some old volume loss in this region before, but the acute space-occupying process on the L has obstructed the ventricle and incarcerated its temporal horn in the middle cranial fossa (b – closed arrow).

A similar CSF-density area is seen on the L (b – open arrow) and from its location probably represents a smaller, obstructed L temporal horn tip.

In addition, there is a strip of low density parenchyma, involving both grey and white matter and the posteromedial aspect of the L temporal lobe. This pattern suggests the anatomic distribution of the PCA. Why would the patient have both a frontal haematoma and a PCA infarct? This could occur if uncal herniation trapped the PCA, which review confirms. This emphasizes the severity of the acute brain swelling. Observation of the main abnormalities has directed the search intelligently for the more subtle pathology.

Inspection of the extracerebral spaces shows extensive fresh blood in the subarachnoid space, outlining the brainstem and filling the pentagonal suprasellar cistern as well as the distorted, gaping R Sylvian fissure (c – asterisk). However, there is also a fresh L subdural haematoma, which has lifted the cortical surface of the L hemisphere away from the calvarium along a broad front, adding to the sulcal compression.

Gravity shows blood in the R occipital horn as well.

This is a mixed acute-on-chronic process, dominated by extensive acute haemorrhage. The epicentre of the process is near the posterior L frontal lobe. In view of the previous aneurysm surgery and this constellation of catastrophic abnormalities, rupture of a second, unsuspected aneurysm is most likely.

Diagnosis

Ruptured aneurysm.

Applying the principles

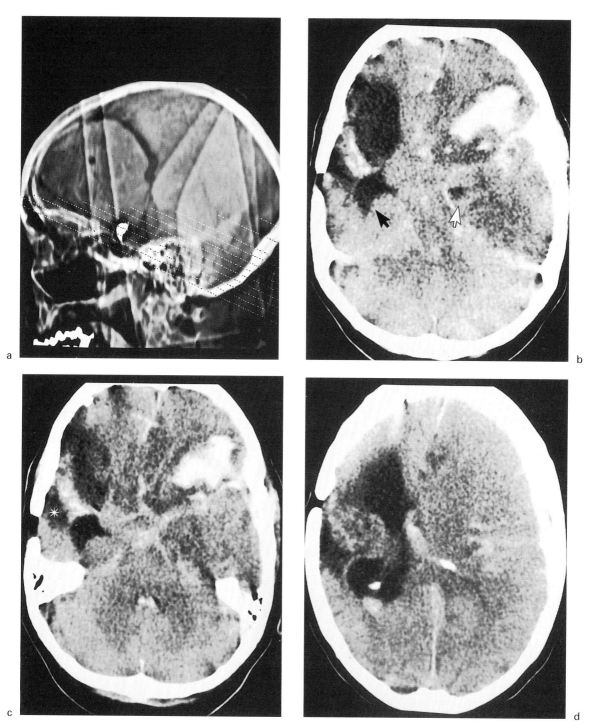

Fig. 8.1

Case
2

Fig. 8.2 (a–b)

Clinical problem

This 67-year-old Australian farmer had a long history of a painless scalp swelling.

Image analysis

Two enhanced scans show a focal transcranial process which has a round shape. It has smoothly eroded bone outwards and bulges into the extracranial soft tissues. The transcranial growth pattern favours an extra-axial process.

It is single and space occupying, with ventricles and sulci being smaller than expected at 67, due to competition for intracranial volume. The smooth bone erosion and lack of vasogenic oedema suggest however an indolent non-aggressive lesion which could even be developmental.

Its internal physical characteristics are heterogeneous to the point of being bizarre. It is predominantly of low density, suggesting fluid, but it is not as low in density as the CSF. Focal areas and the rim have enhanced in a reasonably orderly fashion.

Diagnosis

Intradiploic dermoid (with built-in viewing port!).

Applying the principles

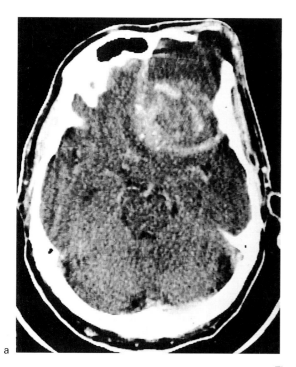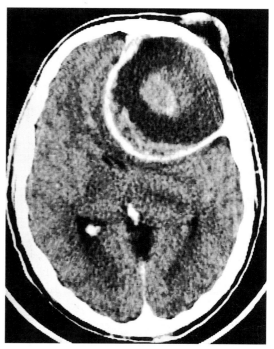

a
b

Fig. 8.2

Case

3

Fig. 8.3 (a–d)

Clinical problem

This 80-year-old man presented in an acute confusional state.

Image analysis

(a) is unenhanced; (b) and (c) enhanced.

There is a well circumscribed R frontal mass which is slightly hyperdense to brain on plain scans and which enhances with IV contrast. There are scattered areas of low attenuation within the tumour.

The mass is sharply marginated, especially posteromedially, with clear demarcation from the oedematous underlying brain. The mass is D-shaped on the direct coronal scan. Its epicentre relates to the anterior cranial fossa floor. The lesion is thus considered extra-axial in location.

It has caused focal erosion of the R greater wing of sphenoid (arrow) "in b" and is beginning to bulge into the R middle cranial fossa. The finer coronal slice windowed on bone (d) shows extensive smooth thinning of the roof of the R orbit, in keeping with the presence of a long-standing mass. Despite some slightly atypical features the most likely diagnosis is meningioma.

Diagnosis

R frontal meningioma with focal myxoid change at surgery. The demonstration that this was an extra-axial mass was important in deciding management for this patient.

Applying the principles

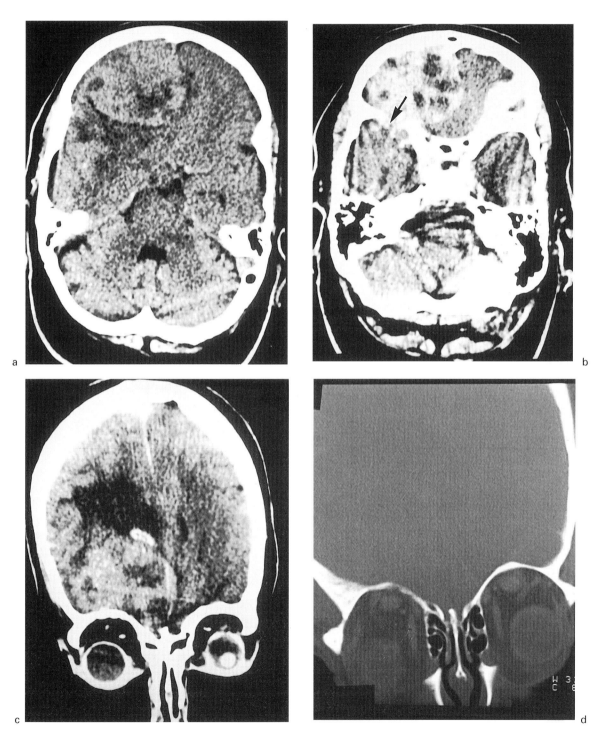

Fig. 8.3

Case

4

Fig. 8.4 (a–d)
(Scout film plus 3 unenhanced images including a bone setting)

Clinical problem

This 70-year-old lady presented with a transient ischaemic attack.

Image analysis

The scout film shows destruction of the pituitary fossa. This is confirmed on the axial slices. Intravenous contrast could not be used due to patient allergy.

The petrous tips have been cleanly amputated bilaterally. Primary pituitary tumour is a reasonable first diagnosis. Chordoma enters the differential diagnosis but one might expect more aggressive destruction and perhaps some calcification. Other skull base tumours such as plasmacytoma should also be considered.

Review of the scout film for ancillary information gives the answer: there are multiple lytic lesions in the vault.

Diagnosis

Multiple myeloma with large skull base deposit. (The patient developed multiple cranial nerve signs soon after her initial presentation).

Applying the principles

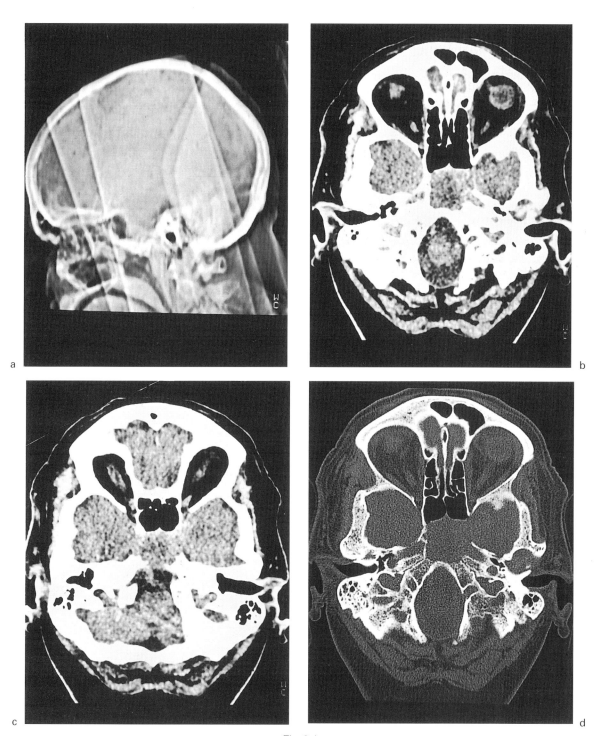

a

b

c

d

Fig. 8.4

Case
5

Fig. 8.5 (a–b) (+C)

Clinical problem

This 47-year-old man had had a R frontal oligodendroglioma removed 12 years before with radiotherapy at that time. Recent deterioration in mental state.

Image analysis

(a) shows local post-operative atrophy with ballooning of the R frontal horn. A surgical clip is present, causing streak artefact. No abnormal mass or tumour enhancement is shown, but there is dural enhancement which is present somewhat later after therapy than one might expect.

(b) confirms the extensive surgical changes.

So far this all looks fairly old, with atrophic features predominating. But where is the R Sylvian fissure? Closer inspection fails to reveal it or normal grey–white differentiation around it. Here a single observation of space-occupation, prior to the development of ventricular compression or midline shift, has swung the diagnosis away from the consequences of therapy to the suspicion of recurrent tumour.

Diagnosis

Recurrent infiltrating low-grade oligodendroglioma confirmed on MR and at surgery.

Applying the principles

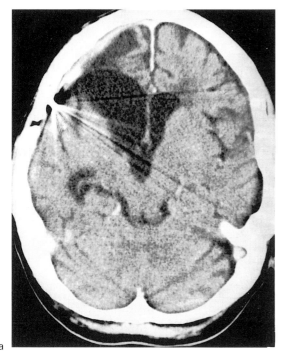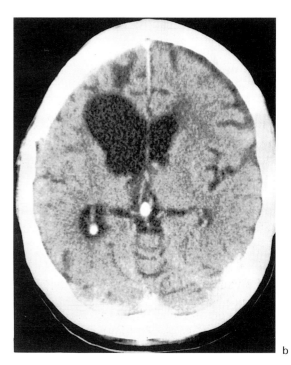

a

b

Fig. 8.5

Glossary

Abbreviations

Anatomy

ACA, MCA, PCA	= Anterior, middle and posterior cerebral arteries
CSF	= Cerebrospinal fluid
LV	= Lateral ventricle
PICA	= Posterior inferior cerebellar artery
V3, V4	= Third, fourth ventricles

Pathology

AGCC	= Agenesis of corpus callosum
AIDS	= Acquired immunodeficiency syndrome
HSE	= Herpes simplex encephalitis
PML	= Progressive multifocal leukoencephalopathy

Physics

+/− C	= With or without intravenous contrast
C	= Centre of window
Hu	= Hounsfield units
ROI	= Region of interest
W	= Photographic window

Index